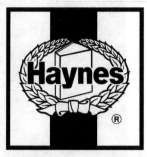

The Man
Manual

Dr Ian Banks

Models Covered
Various, all shapes, sizes and colours

(3931 - 128)

ABCDE
FGHIJ
KLMNO
PQR

© Ian Banks 2002

ISBN 1 85960 931 7

British Library Cataloguing in Publication Data
A catalogue record for this book is available from the British Library.

Printed by **J H Haynes & Co Ltd,**
Sparkford, Yeovil, Somerset BA22 7JJ, England.

Haynes Publishing
Sparkford, Yeovil, Somerset BA22 7JJ, England

Haynes North America, Inc
861 Lawrence Drive, Newbury Park, California 91320, USA

Editions Haynes
4, Rue de l'Abreuvoir
92415 COURBEVOIE CEDEX, France

Haynes Publishing Nordiska AB
Box 1504, 751 45 UPPSALA, Sverige

Contents

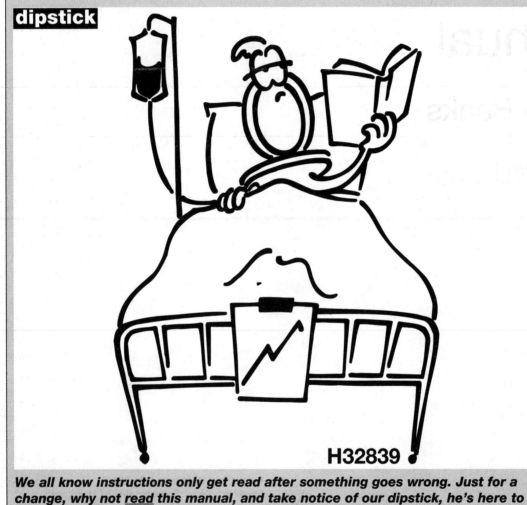

dipstick

H32839

We all know instructions only get read after something goes wrong. Just for a change, why not <u>read</u> this manual, and take notice of our dipstick, he's here to provide tips, but mainly to show you just how NOT to do it.

Contents

A man manual is a pretty obvious idea, but only after somebody has thought of it. A workshop worth of people put this particular model together. Concept design must go to Stuart Mayell and Rob Cohen. For sheer enthusiasm and traction, Mark Sudwell was more than just torque. James Campbell made dipsticks come to life while Ian Mauger made some sense of the exercise. Bob Gann gave support on line from NHS Direct, Simon Gregory was referred to for a second opinion and Matthew Minter turned a run-about into a classic. If you ever find yourself in the pits, these guys will get you out of them.

Note: *The similarities between NHS Direct On Line and sections of this book are no coincidence. It is with grateful thanks that the Haynes workshop team acknowledge the invaluable contribution from the NHS Healthcare Guide and Encyclopaedia. For more information see NHS Direct On line.*

The Man Manual has been produced in association with the Men's Health Forum and sponsored by an unrestricted educational grant from Lilly ICOS.

The Author and the Publisher have taken care to ensure that the advice given in this edition is current at the time of publication. The Reader is advised to read and understand the instructions and information material included with all medicines recommended, and to consider carefully the appropriateness of any treatments. The Author and the Publisher will have no liability for adverse results, inappropriate or excessive use of the remedies offered in this book or their level of effectiveness in individual cases. The Author and the Publisher do not intend that this book be used as a substitute for medical advice. Advice from a medical practitioner should always be sought for any symptom or illness.

HAYNES PUBLISHING: MORE THAN JUST MANUALS

Haynes Publishing Group is the worldwide market leader in the production and sale of car and motorcycle repair manuals. Every vehicle manual is based on a complete strip-down and rebuild in our workshops. This approach, reflecting thoroughness and attention to detail, is integral to all our publications.

The Group publishes many other DIY titles as well as an extensive array of books about motor sport, vehicles and transport in general. Through its subsidiary Sutton Publishing the Group has also extended its interests to include history books.

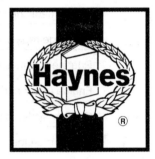

LILLY ICOS LLC: A PARTNERSHIP FOR NEW SOLUTIONS

Lilly ICOS is a joint venture combining the expertise of two leading companies:

Eli Lilly and Company Limited - one of the world's leading pharmaceutical companies. Lilly has a huge commitment to research & development and has been behind many of the most innovative pharmaceuticals, including the world's first commercially available insulin product.

ICOS, located in Washington USA, is a company at the forefront of the biotechnology revolution, with expertise in molecular, cellular and structural biology.

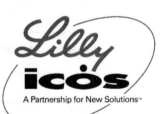

MHF

The Men's Health Forum is a charity that aims to improve men's health in England and Wales through:

Research and policy development
Professional training
Providing information services
Stimulating professional and public debate
Working with MPs and Government
Developing innovative and imaginative projects
Collaborating with the widest possible range of interested organisations and individuals
Organising the annual National Men's Health Week

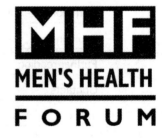

Dedication

The Man Manual is dedicated to the memory of Ian Mauger, Business Development Director for Haynes Publishing, who saw the potential of the book and without whom the project would never have begun. Reading the early drafts of the text prompted Ian to consult his GP about a digestive problem; tragically this proved to be due to oesophageal cancer and despite a brave and inspiring fight he died in July 2002.

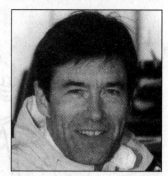

Haynes manuals are truly iconic to British men young and old. For more than 40 years the famous step by step guides and jargon-free information have helped us love and care for our treasured motors.

Men trust Haynes, so I think it is an act of genius to use this famous format to talk to men about their bodies and their health.

For too long men have not been proactive in seeking information about their health. This lack of knowledge is a potent fuel when mixed with fear and embarrassment, and stops men from coming forward with their symptoms – a major reason why treatable conditions such as diabetes, prostate cancer and impotence often remain untreated, causing misery to millions.

This manual sits in pole position to change this, and I am delighted to endorse it. Haynes and the Men's Health Forum have worked tirelessly with sponsor Lilly ICOS to cement this radical partnership and make a real difference.

So a place on the podium to all those who worked to get this manual past the chequered flag, and victory wreaths to you the reader – you've made the first step towards championship health.

Gentlemen, start your engines…..

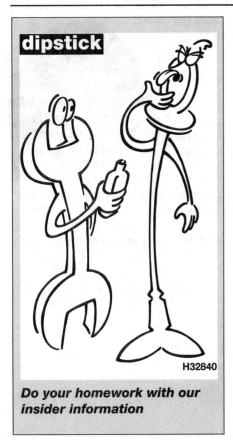

dipstick

H32840

Do your homework with our insider information

Write down your symptoms before you see your doctor:
• It is easy to forget the most important things during the examination. Doctors home-in on important clues. When did it start? How did it feel? Did anyone else suffer as well? Did this ever happen before? What have you done about it so far? Are you on any medicines at present?

Arrive informed:
• Check out the net for information before you go to the surgery. There are thousands of sites on health but many of them are of little real use. Click on NHS Direct as a start, or look in the reference section at the back of this book for up-to-date and accurate information.

Ask questions:
• If a mechanic stuck his head into the bonnet of your car you would most certainly want to know what he intended. This doctor is about to lift the lid on your body. Don't be afraid to ask questions about what a test will show, how a particular treatment works, and when you should come back. After all, its your man machine.

Avoid asking for night visits unless there is a good reason:
• Calling your GP after you have 'suffered' all day at work will antagonise a doctor who thinks personal health should come before convenience. If you put money before their quality of family life don't be surprised if you are asked to come to the surgery the following morning.

Don't beat around the bush:
• If you have a lump on your testicles say so. With an average of only seven minutes for each consultation its important to get to the point. There is a real danger of going to your doctor with erection problems and coming out with a prescription for piles cream.

Your Health is a partnership:
• Now is the time to convince your family doctor to take a serious look at men's health, in particular yours. No screening system exists at present but nothing prevents you from asking for a consultation to examine risk factors. A strong family history of conditions such as heart disease, diabetes, cancer or eye problems like glaucoma should prompt some basic tests.

Listen to what the doctor says:
• If you don't understand, say so. It helps if they write down the important points. Most people pick up less than half of what their doctor has told them.

Have your prescription explained:
• Three items on a scrip will cost you as much as a half decent tyre. Ask whether you can buy any of them from the chemist. Make sure you know what they are all for. Some medicines clash badly with alcohol. Even one pint of beer with some popular antibiotics will make you feel very ill. Mixing antidepressants and alcohol can be fatal. Are there any side effects you should look out for? Many prescribed medicines cause erectile dysfunction (impotence).

If you want a second opinion say so:
• Ask for a consultant appointment by all means but remember you are dealing with a person with feelings and not a computer. Compliment him for his attention first but then explain your deep anxiety.

Flattery will get you anywhere:
• Praise is thin on the ground these days. An acknowledgment of a good effort, even if not successful, will be remembered.

Be courteous with all the staff:
• Receptionists are not dragons trying to prevent you seeing a doctor. Practice nurses increasingly influence your treatment. General practice is a team effort and you will get the best out of it by treating all its members with respect.

Be prepared to complain:
• If possible see your doctor first and explain what is annoying you. Family doctors now have an 'in-house' complaints system, and most issues are successfully resolved at this level. If you are still not satisfied you can take it to a formal hearing.

Trust your doctor:
• There is a difference between trust and blind faith. Your health is a partnership between you and your doctor where you are the majority stakeholder.

Change your GP with caution:
• Thousands of people change their doctor each year. Most of them have simply moved house. You do not need to tell your family doctor if you wish to leave their practice. Your new doctor will arrange for all your notes to be transferred. The whole point of general practice is to build up a personal insight into the health of you and your family. A new doctor has to start almost from scratch.

Don't be afraid to ask to see your notes:

• You have the right to see what your doctor writes about you. Unfortunately doctors' language can be difficult to understand. Latin and Greek are still in use although on the decline. Doctors use abbreviations in your notes. Watch out for:

a) *TATT: An abbreviation for Tired All The Time.*

b) *TCA SOS: To Call Again if things get worse. Most illnesses are self-limiting. A couple of weeks usually allows nature to sort things out.*

c) *RV: Review. Secretaries will automatically arrange a subsequent appointment.*

d) *PEARLA: Pupils Equal and Reacting to Light and Accommodation. A standard entry on a casualty sheet to show that your brain is functioning.*

e) *RTA: Road Traffic Accident.*

f) *FROM: Full Range Of Movement at a joint.*

g) *SOB: Short Of Breath. If this comes on after walking in from the waiting room it turns into SOBOE – On Exercise.*

h) *AMA/CMA: Against Medical Advice/Contrary Medical Advice: You went home despite medical advice not to do so.*

i) *DNA: Did Not Attend. You didn't turn up for your appointment.*

j) *SUPRATENTORIAL: If your doctor thinks you are deluding yourself over your symptoms and its really all in your head, he might think the problem lies above (supra) your tentorium. Rarely used these days.*

k) *HYSTERIA: A dangerous diagnosis. In essence your doctor believes you are possibly over-dramatising the situation. Rarely used these days.*

l) *C_2H_5OH: The chemical formula for alcohol. Your doctor probably believes alcohol plays a role in your problem. Rarely used these days.*

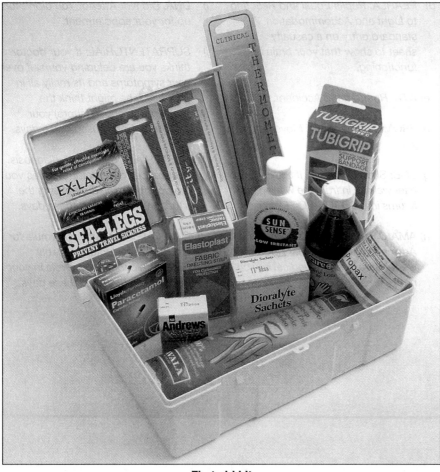

First aid kit

Minor illnesses or accidents can happen at any time so it's worth being prepared. It makes sense to keep some first aid and simple remedies in a safe place in the house to cover most minor ailments and accidents. The picture shows an example of a well stocked and maintained kit. Ask your pharmacist for advice on which products are best.

- Painkillers.
- Mild laxatives.
- Anti-diarrhoeal, rehydration mixture.
- Indigestion remedy, eg antacids.
- Travel sickness tablets.
- Sunscreen – SPF15 or higher.
- Sunburn treatment.
- Tweezers, sharp scissors.
- Thermometer.
- A selection of plasters, cotton wool, elastic bandages and assorted dressings.

Remember:
- Keep the medicine chest in a secure, locked place, out of reach of small children.
- Do not keep in the bathroom as the damp will soon damage the medicines and bandages.
- Always read the instructions and use the right dose.
- Watch expiry dates – don't keep or use medicines past their sell-by date.

Chapter 1
Roadside repairs (first aid)

Contents

1 First aid

Accidents account for greatest loss of life amongst young men. Car crashes, sports injuries, industrial accidents and dodgy DIY are all major causes of injury and death.

Having someone around with first aid knowledge can make the difference. Anyone can learn these simple but often life saving techniques.

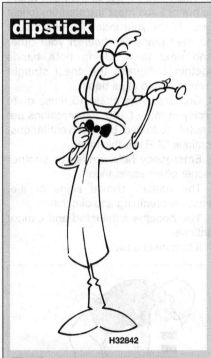

The best way to gain new skills is from an expert. Do a course and look like Dr Kildare in an emergency. Contact the St John Ambulance or the British Heart Foundation

2 Myths of first aid

Below are some commonly asked questions and answers:

You will be successfully sued if you look after someone and they think you were negligent:
• **Wrong:** The good Samaritan principle should keep you safe from successful litigation in most cases. You are only expected to be able to do what any other non-medically trained person could do.

Men should not look after injured women in case they are accused of sexual harassment:
• **Wrong:** Common-sense prevails. Do what you need to do to save her life. If another woman is present, use her to chaperone. Explain out loud what you are doing even if she appears unconscious, it also helps to calm onlookers.

People always faint when they see all the blood:
• **Wrong.** If you know what you need to do and you get on with it you will probably not faint.

You will catch HIV if you perform mouth to mouth resuscitation on someone with AIDS:
• **Wrong:** Although there is a small theoretical risk, the chances of becoming infected are extremely small.

First aid makes no difference. Getting them to hospital takes precedence:
• **Wrong:** It is vital to get professional help as soon as possible but ambulance drivers generally like to pick up live people on the way to casualty. A person can lose all their blood from a serious wound in a relatively short space of time. You can save someone's life before the ambulance even arrives. After one hour, the so called 'Golden Hour', a person's fate is more or less sealed. You make the difference in the equation.

A little knowledge is a dangerous thing:
• **Wrong:** This is usually quoted by people who would rather not bother. So long as you stick to what you know and use common sense it is unlikely you will make the situation any worse.

Doing something is always better than doing nothing:
• **Wrong.** People with no idea can be a danger to your health. Giving a badly injured person alcohol might bring their colour back but if they're bleeding it could kill them. Get trained.

3 It seemed like a good idea (common mistakes)

We all carry ideas on what to do in an emergency. Most of them come from the movies.

Don't give a casualty anything to eat or drink.
• If a person is unable to swallow properly, for example after a stroke or head injury, you could choke them, and if they need surgery the anaesthetist would not thank you.

Don't leave an unconscious or drunk person lying on their back.
• Vomit or even their own tongue could block their airway. Stay with them, but shout to attract help or if possible use a mobile telephone.

Don't be afraid to call the emergency services.
• If you are not sure whether you are out of your depth you probably are. Send two people to phone at the same time. Get one to return and let you know what's happening, and tell one to stay and direct the ambulance.

Don't use a tourniquet.
• Once a tourniquet is released all the debris in the blood blocks up the kidneys. Instead press firmly on the wound to stop the bleeding.

Don't put yourself in danger.
• If it goes wrong the emergency services have two casualties to deal with. Check your surroundings first for falling rocks, fumes, cars, live electricity, etc.

4 Cardio-pulmonary resuscitation (kiss of life)

Simply reading how to perform cardio-pulmonary-resuscitation (CPR) is like expecting to be able to drive a Porsche after reading the workshop manual. You need to be trained before having to do it for real.

1 Take a moment to check you are not in danger. Look around and make sure you will be safe to help.
2 Try and get the man to respond, talk to him, gently squeeze his shoulder. Look for even small movements and listen carefully. If you get no response

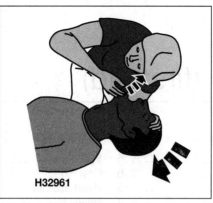

4.5 Clear the airway by extending the head backwards

shout for help. Dial 999/112 from a mobile or landline.
3 Check the ABC (that's Airway, Breathing and Circulation):
4 First clear the airway (A). Tip the head backwards extremely gently, and clear anything out of the mouth.
5 Listen carefully for breathing (B). Look along the chest for movement and place your ear and cheek close to the injured man's mouth to listen and feel for breathing.
6 If the patient is not breathing then start the first part of CPR (cardio-pulmonary resuscitation), the so-called Kiss of Life.
7 Pinch the man's nose, take a deep breath and then place your lips over the man's mouth, trying to create a seal. Then steadily blow over a period of two seconds (this is one 'ventilation'). Watch to see the chest wall rise. If there is no movement then readjust the airway and try again. You can attempt this five times. Once it works make sure you get two full breaths in.
8 Now you need to check the patient's circulation (C). Check for a pulse (using

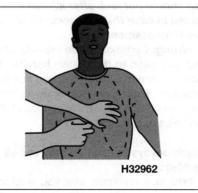

4.10A Correct position of hands for chest compressions

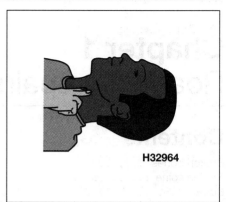

4.8 Checking for a pulse at the artery in the neck

your first two fingers) at the artery in the neck, found on the left side of the neck, just under the chin. Take up to 10 seconds to check this properly, and look at the man's colour, temperature and generally any signs of life.
9 If there is no signs of circulation perform the second part of CPR, chest compressions or heart massage.
10 First locate the right hand position. Put your middle finger at the point where the bottom ribs meet the sternum (chest bone). Place your index finger above it and then place the heel of your other hand next to it. Using both hands together compress the chest straight down to a third of its depth.
11 Compress the chest 15 times quite quickly (a rate of 100 compressions per minute), followed by two ventilations. Continue CPR like this until:
• Emergency help arrives or another rescuer offers assistance.
• The patient shows signs of life. Reassess breathing and circulation.
• You become exhausted and cannot continue.
• It becomes unsafe.

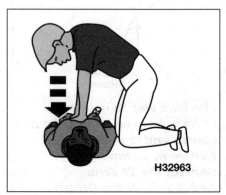

4.10B Keep arms straight with each thrust

5 Broken bones

Bones contain blood vessels and nerves. A fracture is painful, more so if the broken ends are sticking into flesh. Follow these simple rules:

1 Tell the injured person to keep still. Steady and support the limb with your hands.

2 Cover any wounds with a dressing or clean non fluffy material, eg shirt. Press as hard as required to stop the bleeding. Bandage the dressing onto the limb.

3 If a leg is broken, tie both legs together with a piece of wood or rolled up magazines between them. Tie the knees and ankles together first then closer to the broken bone.

4 Suspected broken arms or collar bones should be supported by fastening the arm on the affected side to the body.

5 Always check that the hands or feet are warm and colour returns after squeezing a nail. If not, loosen the bandages a little.

6 Swelling can tighten bandages so check every fifteen minutes.

6 Broken spine

A broken neck or spine will not necessarily kill or paralyse you, but if you suspect a broken spine it is essential you follow these simple rules.

1 Do not move the person unless there is imminent danger within the area. If they must be moved, always support the head on each side with gentle but firm pulling and use a number of people to lift in as many places as possible. If possible use a flat piece of wood to carry him while still supporting his head.

2 Reassure the person and tell him not to move. Steady the head with hands on either side of the ears.

3 Get helpers to place rolled blankets or coats around the sides to stop him rolling.

4 Dial 999 or 112 and explain what has happened.

5 Continue to check his breathing while you wait for help.

7 Dislocated joints

Dislocating any joint can damage surrounding nerves, blood vessels, and ligaments. Trying to force the joint back into place can make this ten times worse. Dislocated shoulders are common because it is a relatively lax joint. Horrendous damage can be done by well meaning offers to 'pop it back in'.

1 Simply support the arm against the front of the body and get him to casualty. Don't give him anything to eat or drink as he may need a general anaesthetic.

8 Burns

1 Cool the burn area with cold water. This can take 10 minutes. Send someone for the ambulance if the burn is severe (greater in size than the size of their own palm).

2 Remove watches, bracelets or anything which will cause constriction once the flesh begins to swell. This includes shoes and necklaces.

3 **Don't** remove clothes if they are sticking to the skin.

4 Cover the burn area with light non-fluffy material.

5 Don't apply creams or burst any blisters.

6 With severe burns there will be a rapid loss of fluid from the blood system with a loss of blood pressure. Lay him down and raise his legs. This helps keep blood available for the vital organs as well as the heart, brain, kidney and lungs.

9 Choking

It takes surprisingly little to choke a person. Here's what to do if you see someone choking:

1 Check inside his mouth. If you can see the offending obstruction pull it out. If you can't see it, bend him over and use the flat of your hand to slap him firmly on the back between his shoulder blades five times.

2 If all this fails, go for the Heimlich manoeuvre (the abdominal thrust).

3 Stand behind the person. Put both arms around his waist and interlock your hands.

4 Pull sharply upwards below the ribs. Try five times and go back to number one.

10 Eye injury

Eyes are amazingly tough. Blows from blunt instruments, such as a squash ball, cause extensive damage to the surrounding bone but the eye usually remains intact. Penetrating injuries are a different matter. Flakes of steel from a chisel struck with a hammer travel at the speed of sound. That's significantly faster than the blink of an eye.

1 Lay him on his back and examine the eye. Only wash the eye if there is no obvious foreign body stuck to the eye and it has no open wound.

2 Place a loose pad over the eye and bandage.

3 Take him to hospital.

11 Heart attacks

Heart disease is the single biggest killer of men so you are likely to see it happen at some time. Modern treatment can significantly improve chances of survival if you can get him to hospital quickly. Recognise what's going on. Central chest pain can move upwards to the throat or arms, usually the left arm.

1 Fear causes the release of adrenaline which makes the heart beat faster, increasing the pain, so talk calmly and reassure.

2 Call for an ambulance.

3 If they normally take a tablet or oral spray for chest pain, let them do so.

4 Sit them down but don't force them to lie down if they don't want to.

5 If you would like to know more, look

1

in the Contacts section at the back of this manual, or contact:

British Heart Foundation
14 Fitzhardinge Street, London W1H 6DH
020 7935 0185
www.bhf.org.uk.

12 Heavy bleeding

1 Lay them down. Bleeding from a vein is generally slow and simply pressing a cloth against the wound and raising the affected limb above the level of the heart will stop the bleeding. Get him to hospital.
2 Arterial bleeds can be seriously different. It's hard to miss when it happens. The blood is bright red and comes out in spurts with each heart beat.
3 Press a cloth against the wound and hold it down firmly. If you have to leave them, secure it to the wound with a shirt or towel.
4 Raise their arms and legs to keep the blood pressure up. Some seepage will occur but you may save their life. Get them to hospital.

13 Do the knowledge

The principles of First Aid are easy when explained by an expert on a training course. Whether you end up reassuring an elderly relative after a fall, or saving a choking child, the sense of reward is amazing. The following charities offer courses, why not give them a call today:

British Heart Foundation,
14 Fitzhardinge Street,
London,
W1H 6DH.
020 7935 0185
www.bhf.org.uk

St John Ambulance,
27 St. John's Lane,
London,
EC1M 4BU.
0870-010 4950
www.sja.org.uk

dipstick

H32841

Don't be a Dipstick, get trained.

Chapter 2
Routine maintenance (staying healthy)

Contents

1 Ageing

The natural human life-span appears to be about 100 years although this can vary enormously across the globe. Even within Europe men live different lengths

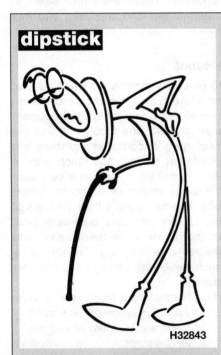

dipstick

H32843

Ageing is one thing that comes to us all, although a regular body service will help keep you running like a Rolls Royce

of time depending on their country and environment.

The bodily and mental changes that occur with ageing usually cause a general improvement and increasing power, both of body and mind, up to about the mid-20s. After that, in most men, there is a gradual decline.

Symptoms

1 There are some generally common facets to the ageing process which include:
a) *Loss of muscle power.*
b) *Deterioration in efficiency of the nervous system.*
c) *Loss of hair colour.*
d) *Decreased skin elasticity with wrinkling and sagging of the skin.*
e) *Thinning of the skin.*
f) *Brittleness of the bones.*
g) *Hardening and narrowing of the arteries.*
h) *Damage to the lenses of the eyes (cataract).*
l) *Poorer recall of memorised facts.*

Causes

2 A number of things make ageing worse, including:
a) *Unhealthy diet.*
b) *Reduced or lack of exercise for body and mind.*
c) *Smoking.*
d) *Substance abuse, including alcohol.*
e) *Excessive exposure to sunlight.*
3 All of these can be modified. The earlier the better.
4 It's also worth keeping an eye out for

warning signs. Even as we get older the best way to stay healthy is to catch problems early. Warning signs of dangerous changes include:
a) *A new, changed or persisting cough.*
b) *Blood in your sputum.*
c) *Black or blood stained stools (motions).*
d) *Any persistent change in your bowel habit.*
e) *Indigestion coming on for the first time in later life.*
f) *Difficulty in swallowing possibly with food returning to your mouth undigested.*
g) *Blood in your vomit.*
h) *Urine or semen with blood stains.*
i) *Any obvious change in a coloured skin spot, mole or wart.*
j) *Any wound or sore that fails to heal in a month.*
k) *Hoarseness or loss of voice, without obvious cause.*
l) *Unexplained weight loss.*

Action

5 Eat less to maintain a normal, low-end-of-range body weight. Avoid saturated fats.
6 Exercise to the point of breathlessness at least three times a week.
7 Stop smoking.
8 Take alcohol in moderation. Aim for no more than 3-4 units of alcohol per day, hopefully less.
9 Have regular blood pressure checks.
10 Take your hobbies seriously, involve others.
11 Make an appointment to see your GP.

2

2 Healthy living

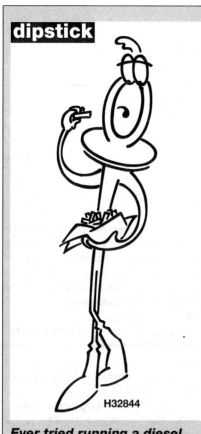

dipstick

H32844

Ever tried running a diesel engine on petrol? Men need the right fuel too

1 Life is for living and it would be much more pleasant if we were all healthier and lived longer to enjoy it. Simple things can make a big difference and don't mean a complete change in the way you live. Here are some tips on how to stay healthy and live longer, without worrying about it.

Eating for pleasure and health

2 Being overweight is on the increase, particularly in men. We know this can increase your risk from heart disease so cutting down on fatty food, especially animal fats, makes sense. Simply grilling food rather than frying will significantly reduce the amount of fat you are eating.

3 Some foods are known to reduce your risk from many illness and possibly even cancer yet are cheap and taste good. Fruit supplies both vitamins and fibre and can replace sweets for children, especially as a 'treat' or reward. Aim for around five servings of fruit or vegetables each day. (One serving is roughly 1 piece of fruit, 1 dessert bowl of salad, 1 glass of fruit juice or 2 tablespoonfuls of vegetables.)

4 Try gradually cutting down on salt with your food. You'll be surprised how little you need after getting used to less. It will protect you from high blood pressure.

5 Fish, especially the oily varieties such as mackerel or sardines are loaded with special oils which actually protect your heart. Bread, especially wholemeal types, potatoes and pasta are all great forms of carbohydrate which provide energy and should be the main part of the meal. Enjoy your food and go for as wide variety as possible.

In a puff of smoke

6 The more we look at smoking and health the more we know that cigarettes are the single greatest killer in our society. Over 300 people die every day from smoking related diseases. Smoking 25 cigarettes a day increases your risk of lung cancer by 25 times and doubles your chances of heart disease.
  a) *Get someone to give up with you and name the day to start.*
  b) *One day at a time is the best plan, but reward yourself each day by putting the money normally spent on cigarettes in a jar.*
  c) *Tell people in the pub or at work that you are trying to stop. These days they will understand and support you.*
  d) *Get rid of all the tobacco stuff in the house like ashtrays, lighters and matches.*
  e) *See your pharmacist, GP or practice nurse about nicotine replacement which will help ease the cravings.*

7 Go for it. You've only your cough to lose in the long run!

Are you active?

8 Most people think they are more active than they actually are. Even a small amount of moderate activity will help protect you from heart disease, still the greatest single cause of death in the UK. Aim to exercise until the point of breathlessness at least three times a week. You don't need to buy expensive machines or even go to gyms or leisure centres.
  a) *Take the stairs instead of the lift.*
  b) *Get off the bus one stop early and walk briskly.*
  c) *Play with the children. Being a 'horse' for them gets your heart pumping.*
  d) *Climb briskly up the house stairs.*
  e) *If possible cycle rather than take the bus or use the car. Most towns are making special tracks for cyclists.*

Sexual health

9 The UK has the highest rate of teenage pregnancies in Europe. At the same time sexually transmitted disease is on the increase. Using simple protective contraception like male or female condoms would help protect against both pregnancy and infections such as HIV.
• Don't be a dipstick. Always use a condom. They are on sale in supermarkets and chemists, and free from family planning clinics.

Alcohol

10 Relatively recently we found out that moderate drinking for men and women over 40 years can actually help prevent heart disease. The problem is that the message gets confused and there is a temptation to drink too much without realising that this protection is very soon lost as the amount of alcohol consumed rises. Aim for no more than 3-4 units of alcohol per day and preferably less. Alcohol abuse is on the increase and children are drinking heavily at a much earlier age, setting the pattern for later life.

11 1 unit of alcohol is roughly the same as:
  a) *An English measure (25ml) of spirit. Scotland and Northern Ireland use larger measures.*
  b) *Half a pint of normal strength beer.*
  c) *One measure of sherry (50ml).*
  d) *One small glass of wine (100ml).*

12 Some beers are very strong and we all pour out more generous measures at home.

3 Nutrition (eat to beat cancer)

Cancer is not inevitable. Some foods actually help prevent it, according to World Cancer Research Fund (WCRF UK).

What do foods have to do with cancer?

• Most cancers are preventable; as many as 30-40% of all cancer cases can be prevented by the types of food we choose to eat. Some foods – especially those which come from plants – can help protect our bodies against cancer.

What do you mean by a 'plant-based' diet?

• A plant-based diet is one in which the majority of the foods come from plants rather than animals. This does not mean a vegetarian diet but most of each meal and snack will be made up of plant foods, including: vegetables and fruits, starchy foods (such as pasta, bread, potatoes and cereals – like rice, corn and oats) and pulses (peas, beans and lentils).

Why is a plant-based diet so important?

• Eating the recommended five portions of vegetables and fruits each day can reduce cancer risk by up to 20%. Research has shown that eating a wide variety of vegetables, fruits, pulses, cereals and other starchy foods may also help to reduce your risk.

How does weight affect cancer risk?

• Being very overweight can increase your risk of cancer – so not only do you need to eat healthily, you also need to take some form of regular physical activity in order to help maintain a healthy body-weight throughout life.

What does exercise have to do with cancer?

• Physical activity is important at all ages to help prevent you from becoming overweight and in helping to protect you from cancer in general. In addition, research has shown that being physically active can itself reduce your risk of certain cancers – particularly of the colon and breast.

A healthier lifestyle

• Ideas for a healthier lifestyle:

a) Opt for wholegrain bread, brown rice and wholemeal pasta instead of the white varieties.

b) Skip meat occasionally and make a delicious meal from a range of fresh seasonal vegetables, some pasta and a tomato-based sauce.

c) Choose skimmed or semi-skimmed rather than full fat dairy products.

d) Remove all visible fat from meat and take the skin off poultry.

e) Take the stairs rather than the lift or escalator when out and about and get off the bus one stop earlier and walk the rest of the way home.

f) Revitalise yourself by going for a brisk walk at any time of the day – morning, lunchtime or evening.

g) If you smoke, try to stop – call Quitline on 0800 00 22 00.

h) Select fish once or twice a week as a healthy alternative to red meat.

j) Cut down on the amount of alcohol you drink – aim for no more than 3-4 units of alcohol per day, and preferably less.

k) Boost your nutrient intake by cooking vegetables lightly and quickly – cook by steaming, or stir-fry.

l) Use salt sparingly – flavour food with herbs and spices instead.

m) Make sure you get plenty of vitamin C – Brussels sprouts, green peppers, broccoli, strawberries, oranges and grapefruits are all good sources.

n) Eat plenty of carrots, spinach, spring greens, marrow, apricots and peaches – they are all good sources of vitamin A.

More information

• If you would like to know more, look in the Contacts section at the back of this manual, or contact:

World Cancer Research Fund,
19 Harley Street,
London,
W1G 9QJ.
Tel: 020 7343 4200
Web: www.wcrf-uk.org

4 Dietary supplements, vitamins and minerals

1 In the past ten years more men have wanted to take responsibility for their own health, and there has been a greater interest in the role played by diet in maintaining good health. There has also been an increase in the number of health supplements available in the UK.
2 However, the number of products now widely available can be confusing and sometimes the information on the products is often conflicting.

When should you think of taking supplements?

3 Most men do get enough nutrients from their diet, but there will always be some men who have low intakes of one or more nutrients or who have special nutritional or medical needs for particular vitamins or minerals at certain times in their lives.
4 Busy lifestyles mean that men are more inclined to skip meals and grab fast food snacks without giving thought to putting together properly balanced meals, which would provide the right mix of nutrients. Nutrients also be lost from food as a result of poor methods of storage, preparation and cooking. Changing your diet is probably the best and cheapest way of getting the nutrients you need. If this isn't possible, ask your pharmacist for advice on supplements.
5 Some nutrients may be difficult to obtain in adequate quantities from food, and therefore have to be taken as a supplement, e.g. cod liver oil, as a source of vitamin D and omega 3 fatty acids.

How do you know the product is safe?

6 Look at the label, for most vitamins and minerals, Upper Safe Levels have

been established so that you can be made aware of the levels of intake, which are safe. These levels have been established by the health supplement industry, using up to date scientific information.

How quickly do they work?

7 Health supplements are not a 'quick fix'. Generally, the body requires a regular supply of nutrients for metabolism, growth and repair of body tissues, as not all nutrients are stored for any great length of time in the body. If these cannot be obtained through diet, then supplements may be useful.

Can you take more than one supplement?

8 Combining supplements will not normally interfere with the way they work and in some cases may be beneficial. However, certain supplements may interact with each other, for example, there is competition in the gut for the absorption of different minerals and a large dose of one might decrease the absorption of another. A multivitamin and/or mineral product is best therefore for all-round supplementation because it delivers nutrients in the right balance. For detailed information/clarification before combining supplements, you should speak to your pharmacist or the manufacturer for advice.

Men on special diets

9 This category may include vegetarians and vegans, because there are some micronutrients which occur mainly in animal products. If you are on a vegetarian diet you need to make sure that you take adequate amounts of vitamin B12, vitamin D, Calcium, Iron and Zinc in your diet. If you are someone who is on a restrictive diet because of a medical condition, you may also benefit from supplementation.

10 Everyone should aim to eat a varied and balanced diet to obtain their nutritional needs, avoiding too many fatty and sugary foods. Supplements should only be used as a top-up where regular consumption of a balanced diet is not possible.

Drinkers / smokers

11 It is well documented that smoking and excess drinking of alcohol, as well as being bad for other aspects of your health, affect many of the nutrients, which are obtained from diet. In particular, the vitamins and minerals that act as antioxidants or in antioxidant systems are important for smokers. These include: vitamin C; vitamin E; plus selenium and zinc. In fact each cigarette smoked destroys some vitamin C and studies indicate that smokers require twice as much vitamin C as non-smokers. Obviously the best idea is to give up smoking and drink in moderate amounts.

Men 65 +

12 As our bodies age, they become less efficient at absorbing some of the nutrients from our diet making it important to ensure that the right quantities of relevant vitamins and minerals are consumed. For example, as we get older our bodies are less able to absorb iron but Vitamin C can help increase absorption. Vitamin D is important to maintain strong bones and teeth while Vitamin E helps to maintain healthy blood vessels. A varied diet will ensure a supply of these essential vitamins and minerals.

5 Weight

1 More than half of us men are overweight – and the proportion is increasing by about one per cent a year. But it doesn't have to be like this; we don't have to resign ourselves to the slow but steady creep of so-called 'middle-age spread'.

Why bother to lose weight?

2 You'll feel better. As you're able to exert greater control over your body size and shape:

a) *Your self-esteem and self-confidence will rise.*

b) *You'll have more energy. That's because your body won't be using up so much simply carrying itself around.*

c) *Your penis could start to look longer as abdominal fat can conceal up to two inches.*

d) *Your sex drive will increase. As you lose weight, your testosterone levels will start to rise, boosting your libido and improving your fertility.*

e) *You'll snore less. Snorers are generally overweight.*

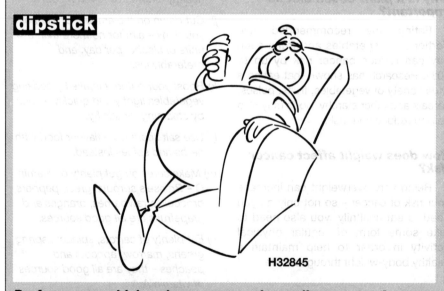

dipstick

H32845

Performance vehicles always carry only small amounts of excess weight. Men, like cars, don't work properly when they're overloaded

f) *You'll live longer. Being overweight is actually a bigger risk factor than smoking for heart disease. Your risk of heart disease, certain cancers, diabetes, gall bladder disease and a range of bone, joint and skin disorders will fall as you lose weight.*

The fat facts

3 Lighter men live longer on average. A man of any age who weighs 11.5 stone and is 5 feet 10 inches tall has a 30% lower risk of dying in any given year than a man of the same height who weighs 16.5 stone.

4 Non-obese men generally have healthier hearts. A man with a body mass index (BMI) of 22 or 23 is about half as likely to suffer from major coronary heart disease as a man with a BMI of over 30. He is also over eight times less likely to develop diabetes.

5 A 20% rise in body weight creates an 86% greater risk of heart disease.

6 Losing weight can lower blood pressure.

7 Obese men are more likely to develop cancer. There's strong evidence linking obesity to an increased risk of colon cancer, especially in men who are also physically inactive.

8 Being overweight increases the risk of arthritis.

Are you overweight?

9 There are three easy ways of working out whether your health could be at risk.

The waist test

10 Your circumference is a good, rough-and-ready indicator of your overall body fat level. Simply stand up and find your natural waist line (it's mid-way between your lowest rib and the top of the hip bone). Place a tape around this line and take a measurement after relaxing your abdomen by breathing out gently. If you measure 37-39.5 inches, you're technically overweight. If your waist tops 40 inches, then you're clinically obese.

The body mass index

11 There are two ways to calculate your body mass index (BMI):

a) *Using pounds and inches. Multiply your weight in pounds by 700 and divide that figure by the square of your height in inches. For example, if you're 68 inches tall and weigh 185 lb, your BMI = 185 x 700 ÷ (68 x 68 = 4624) = 28.*

b) *Using kilograms and metres. Dividing your weight by the square of your height. This means that if you're 1.78 metres tall and weigh 78kg, your BMI = 78 ÷ (1.78 x 1.78 = 3.2) = 24.4.*

12 Ideally, your score should be between 20 and 25 (in fact, a BMI of about 22 is probably best for long-term health); below 20 and you're underweight; between 25 and 30, you're overweight; and if you're above 30, you're obese. This is the standard test used to check whether your weight could cause health problems. It's not so suitable for fit men with loads of muscle, however, since they could seem overweight even though they're actually carrying very little fat.

Tricks of the trade

- *Spicy foods could help boost your metabolic rate, helping you to lose weight. (The metabolic rate is a measure of how quickly your body burns calories to produce energy.) Beware though, Indian takeaway food is high in fat.*

- *Eat different foods. If the body regularly consumes foods with which it's familiar, its metabolic rate is lower than if it has to digest something new.*

- *Use oil-free salad dressings, such as balsamic vinegar or plain lemon juice.*

- *Eat fruit for dessert rather than a cake or pudding. Replace ice-cream with frozen fat-free yoghurt or sorbet.*

- *Keep an emergency supply of low-fat snacks handy to tackle hunger pangs. Apples, pears and medium-ripe bananas are especially good at keeping you feeling fuller.*

- *Take your own lunch to work so you have more control over what you eat.*

- *Don't try to cut out all fats. For a start, you'll never be able to do it unless you become completely obsessive about everything you eat. Second, your body actually needs some fats to function – they carry important vitamins and help produce key hormones.*

- *Eat less food more often.*

- *Always eat a hearty but less fat breakfast.*

- *Eat smaller portions. A good way of doing this is simply to eat off a smaller plate.*

- *Eat more slowly. This will allow time for your body's appetite control mechanism to cut in when you're full, enabling you to avoid a second helping.*

- *Use low-fat margarines instead of butter on bread.*

- *Switch to fat-free or low-fat dairy products. Use semi-skimmed or skimmed milk on your cereal and in your tea or coffee.*

- *When eating meat, trim off any excess fat and remove the skin before eating poultry.*

- *Cook vegetables in stock rather than sautéing them in oil or butter. Have your potatoes baked or boiled but not fried or roasted.*

- *Set yourself a realistic weight target, perhaps something you've weighed in at before, but not too far in the distant past.*

- *Think long-term. A steady loss of 1-2lb a week, or a 1% per week reduction in waist size, is realistic and sustainable.*

2

Height / weight chart – Imperial (height in inches, weight in pounds)

Height	Underweight	Healthy weight	Overweight	Obese
63	up to 113	113 – 141	141 – 169	169 plus
64	up to115	115 – 144	144 – 173	173 plus
65	up to 121	121 – 151	151 – 182	182 plus
66	up to 124	124 – 155	155 – 186	186 plus
67	up to127	127 – 159	159 – 191	191 plus
68	up to 132	132 – 165	165 – 197	197 plus
69	up to 135	135 – 168	168 – 202	202 plus
70	up to 140	140 – 174	174 – 209	209 plus
71	up to143	143 – 178	178 – 214	214 plus
72	up to 147	147 – 184	184 – 221	221 plus
74	up to 155	155 – 194	194 – 233	233 plus
75	up to 159	159 – 199	199 – 238	238 plus

Height / weight chart – metric (height in metres, weight in kilograms)

Height	Underweight	Healthy weight	Overweight	Obese
1.60	up to 51	51 – 64	64 – 77	77 plus
1.63	up to 52	52 – 65	65 – 79	79 plus
1.65	up to 55	55 – 69	69 – 83	83 plus
1.68	up to 56	56 – 70	70 – 84	84 plus
1.70	up to 58	58 – 72	72 – 87	87 plus
1.73	up to 60	60 – 75	75 – 89	89 plus
1.75	up to 61	61 – 76	76 – 92	92 plus
1.78	up to 64	64 – 79	79 – 95	95 plus
1.80	up to 65	65 – 81	81 – 97	97 plus
1.83	up to 67	67 – 84	84 – 100	100 plus
1.88	up to 70	70 – 88	88 – 106	106 plus
1.91	up to 72	72 – 90	90 – 108	108 plus

The waist : hip ratio

13 Measure your waist and hips. (It doesn't matter whether you do this in centimetres or inches.) Measure the circumference of your waist as described in the waist test; your hips should be measured at their widest part.

14 Divide your waist measurement by your hip measurement to get a ratio. For example, if your waist is 90cm and your hips 105cm, the ratio is 0.86. If your ratio is greater than 0.95, you need to lose some weight. This is a particularly useful test because it assesses your fat distribution and calculates whether you have too much around your abdomen.

6 Unexpected weight loss

1 Losing weight, or at least trying to lose weight, is very popular at the moment. This is perfectly reasonable if you are overweight, but there should be a good reason why you are seeing the pounds drop off. A significant loss of weight (over 4.5kg (10lbs) in 10 weeks) for no good reason is not normal. Increasing exercise will decrease your weight so long as you are not eating more than usual. Cutting down on alcohol if you have been drinking too much will also trim your waistline. But if you are losing weight but cannot pin down exactly why, you should be aware of some medical conditions which include weight loss in their list of signs and symptoms.

2 Do you have an increased thirst, pass water more often and feel generally tired? Some hormone deficiencies such as diabetes can cause weight loss with these symptoms. This condition tends to run in families, so if a close relative suffered from diabetes it will increase your risk. A simple test can be performed by your practice nurse.

3 Feeling restless, sweating profusely, feeling weak and having difficulty sleeping may be the signs of a hyperactive thyroid gland, which is producing too much thyroxine. This will cause weight loss by increasing your basic metabolic rate. Again, a simple blood test can check this for you.

4 Some rare infections like tuberculosis and even rarer disorders of the immune system such as AIDS can also cause weight loss. It is possible for your doctor to check for these conditions in a number of ways, including blood tests and X-rays.

5 Persistent diarrhoea with unusually pale stools may mean you are not absorbing your food properly. This may be due to an inflammation of the digestive system. Any marked changes in your bowel habit (how often you pass a motion) or any blood or tar-like substances in your stool, can be caused by inflammation or a tumour. This is not always accompanied by abdominal pain, although if pain is present, there is even more reason to get it checked sooner rather than later.

7 Smoking

1 Lung cancer was rare until tobacco hit the scene. Some things will not go away in a puff of smoke.

2 Lung cancer is the most common type of cancer in men with over 100 new cases per 100,000 men diagnosed each year in the UK. 31% of all deaths from any cancer are from lung cancer. 30,000 men develop it each year.

3 Lung cancer is most common between the ages of 65 and 75; it is relatively rare below the age of 40.

4 Only 8% of people survive lung cancer.

5 The more cigarettes smoked and the younger the age at which smoking started, the greater the risk. Cigar and pipe smokers have a lower chance of developing lung cancer, but their risk is still higher than for non-smokers.

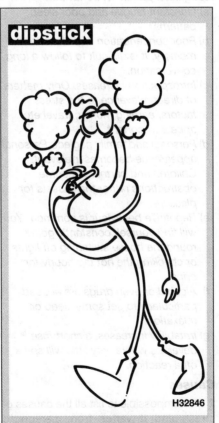

dipstick

Cars with smoking exhausts don't look or smell healthy, and they invariably fail their MOTS

6 Inhalation of tobacco smoke by non-smokers – known as passive smoking – has also been shown to be a risk factor for lung cancer.

Symptoms

7 You should go to your GP if you:
   a) *have a persistent cough.*
   b) *are coughing up blood.*
   c) *have an increasing shortness of breath.*

Causes

8 Smoking causes lung cancer. Even the tobacco companies now accept this simple fact.

Prevention

9 Giving up smoking or better still, not starting in the first place makes sense. Try to get your head around the fact 100 people die every day from smoking.

10 Imagine what you'll miss. Half of all heavy smokers will never reach 70 years of age. Even light smokers only have a 60% chance of survival until the age of 70.

11 There are now four times as many non-smokers as smokers, so you can do it if you really put your mind to it. There is plenty of help available.

Once you're ready to go, produce a quit plan. Here's how to do it

12 Set a day and date to stop. Tell all your friends and relatives, they will support you.

13 Like deep sea diving, always take a buddy. Get someone to give up with you. You will reinforce each other's willpower.

14 Clear the house and your pockets of any packets, papers or matches.

15 One day at a time is better than leaving it open ended.

16 Map out your progress on a chart or calendar. Keep the money saved in a separate container.

17 Chew on a carrot. Not only will it help you do something with your mouth and hands, it also contains beta carotene which inhibits cancer.

18 Ask your friends not to smoke around you. People accept this far more readily than they used to do.

2

Once you've stopped smoking

19 Within 8 hours all of the poisonous carbon monoxide produced by smoking has been washed out of your blood. At the same time the oxygen levels return to normal.

20 Within 24 hours your chances of a heart attack, much higher while smoking, begin to decrease.

21 Within 48 hours the nerve endings destroyed by smoking begin to re-grow. You may well find yourself clearing your lungs better after two smoke-free days. Your sense of smell will become stronger as will your taste. Many people put on weight after stopping smoking for just these reasons, they enjoy their food more.

22 Within 3 days spasm of lung tissue decreases making breathing easier. Lung capacity increases.

23 Within 3 months your circulation has improved, walking becomes easier and even your liver begins to improve. Most of the detoxification of the nasties absorbed from smoke takes place in the liver.

24 Within 5 years your risk of lung cancer has dropped dramatically – some doctors say by up to 50% – and the risk will return to normal within 10 years.

Action

25 See your pharmacist, doctor or practice nurse.

26 Nicotine patches can be obtained through your GP or pharmacist. These can be very successful in easing the craving for nicotine.

27 If you are really determined to quit your GP may offer you a new type of medicine which works in the brain to stop cravings.

28 Get as much help and support as you can. Call self-help groups or organisations like Quit. They'll supply loads of free information and advice.

Further information

29 If you would like to know more, look in the Contacts section at the back of this manual, or contact:

QUIT,
Ground Floor,
211 Old Street, London, EC1V 9NR.
Smokers' Quit-line: 0800 00 22 00
www.quit.org.uk

30 If you can't do it for yourself, do it for your partner or kids.

8 Coping with stress

Life can never be free from some level of stress. It is valuable to produce a better performance in many aspects of our lives. Some people even thrive on stress and will seek it out in the form of dangerous sports or jobs.

We all have different abilities of coping with stress and when it becomes too great it is no longer useful and can become extremely destructive.

Learning to cope with stress and to use it to your advantage is one the great challenges of these stress ridden times. People experience different 'triggers' which make them stressed. Recognising them is the first part of dealing with stress itself.

Symptoms

1 As stress builds up there is a recognised pattern of behaviour.

 a) *Constant fatigue and poor sleep patterns.*

 b) *Poor concentration and short-term memory, it is difficult to follow a long conversation.*

 c) *Introspection increases. Only matters of direct relevance to the stress factors, earning money, travel etc. appear important.*

 d) *Personal and family neglect. Personal appearance becomes irrelevant. Children and partners become obstructions rather than assets for pleasure.*

 e) *Repetitive behaviour is common. You will find yourself constantly going round the house switching off lights or checking the hot tap hourly for drips.*

 f) *Alcohol or even drugs are abused particularly to get some sleep or relaxation.*

 g) *Irritability increases, a short fuse develops where very little will spark off a reaction.*

Causes

2 It is impossible to list all the causes of stress and it varies from person to person.

3 The severest forms of stress are those things over which you have no control – if you have little money and the children need new clothes for instance.

4 Work, school, relationships, money, moving house, cars and so on will all cause stress at some time.

5 Your state of mind and general health will also be a factor in the way stress affects you and your ability to cope with it.

Prevention

6 Remember your stress triggers and when you get caught up in one, use it as a cue to relax.

Complications

7 Stress can affect almost every part of your body.

8 Increases your risk from high blood pressure, stroke, heart disease, digestive problems including peptic ulcers, reduced ability to fight infection.

9 Further harm can come from alcohol or drug abuse in an attempt to cope with stress.

10 It also can affect personal relationships, work and your sex life.

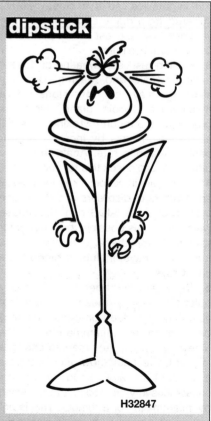

dipstick

H32847

Occasionally we all drive at high revs. Too much of it and you'll blow a gasket

Self care

11 Exercise is a great way to burn off frustration and stress. Strangely, sport which appears stressful can often be the opposite.

12 As an opposite, try peaceful and gentle relaxation techniques such as yoga.

13 Both ways of reducing stress will help sleep patterns without the need to resort to drugs or alcohol.

14 Alcohol and smoking will, at best, provide only short term relief from the effects of stress.

15 At their very worst, in excess they will produce their own problems which will make anything previously causing your stress seem like taking a holiday.

16 You only have one pair of hands. Take jobs in their order of importance instead of trying to do everything at once.

17 Learn to say NO to more work.

18 Conversations require give and take. Stop talking *at* people and listen to what they are saying even if it doesn't seem to fit in with all your worries.

19 Food is important. Eat it, don't just consume it.

20 Talk to people around the table, this is the time to talk about the good things.

21 Share the bath with your partner or young children. Dream and plan holidays.

Action

22 Make an appointment with your GP if you think stress is affecting your overall health.

Further information

23 If you would like to know more, look in the Contacts section at the back of this manual, or contact:

International Stress Management Association,
The Priory Hospital,
Priory Lane, London, SW15 5JJ.

9   Relaxation exercises

Reading a book on how to play the piano will not turn you into a concert pianist. Practice makes perfect, and this is the same with learning how to relax without resorting to alcohol or drugs.

Self Care

1   Make sure you will be alone, it will not help if you are constantly disturbed by requests for another drink of water or to answer a telephone.

2   Either lie on a bed or sit in a chair with your head and arms supported and feet on a stool. Settle down and rid your mind of any thoughts which increase your anxiety.

3   Concentrate on the positive words such as 'relax' or 'unwind'.

4   Gentle music may help but is not essential.

5   Breathe in deeply and hold your breath. Gradually release your breath and, as you do so, let your body sink into the chair or bed.

6   Focusing your tension and release into specific parts of your body can be very effective.

7   Concentrate on your right hand, make it into a fist, tightly clench it, then release it. Do it again. This time concentrate on the tension in your hand and as you release it notice the difference in the way it feels from when it is clenched and when it is relaxed.

8   Do the same with your arms. Flex them and feel the tension build up as you bend your elbow. Imagine you are pulling a heavy weight. Hold the tension for a while and then relax.

9   As you relax breathe out. At the same time reinforce the relaxation by thinking positive thoughts, 'I feel better', 'I am relaxing'.

10 By concentrating on the difference between the relaxed and tensed state of your muscles and linking it to your mental state there will be a logical sequence of reinforcement.

11 Use a set pattern for instance:

a) *Restore the normal state after each action. After tensing a muscle always return to a relaxed state.*

b) *Do you feel the effect? Concentrate on the difference.*

c) *Use a pattern for breathing. Always breathe in as you tense and breathe out as you relax your muscles.*

d) *Even if you think you have completely relaxed a muscle try to release it that bit more.*

e) *Take your time. It will become easier to achieve a state of relaxation more quickly as you become more adept.*

f) *Use positive thoughts to augment your physical activity, 'relax', 'let go' etc.*

g) *Repeat each individual exercise at least twice. You will be surprised at the level of relaxation you will achieve after each repeat.*

h) *Use the same pathway for each part of your body, chest, neck, abdomen, legs and feet. You do not have to adhere rigidly to this system, you will soon find a pattern which suits you best.*

12 Now is the time to reflect on the trivia which can cause such tension and how, with a little practice, they can be seen in their true light.

13 On the other hand you might still feel like pulling all your hair out by the roots, but at least you won't get out of breath.

Further information

14 If you would like to know more, look in the Contacts section at the back of this manual, or contact:

International Stress Management Association,
The Priory Hospital,
Priory Lane,
London,
SW15 5JJ.

MIND (National Association For Mental Health),
Granta House,
15-19 Broadway,
Stratford,
London,
E15 4BQ.

Samaritans,
General Office,
10 The Grove,
Slough, Berks,
SL1 1QP.
0845 790 90 90

2

Chapter 3
Engine (heart and lungs)

Contents

1 Angina (angina pectoris)

Introduction

Angina is a pain or an uncomfortable, often vague feeling of pressure in the chest. It is a symptom that usually lasts only for a few minutes at the most and it will, in most cases, be relieved simply by resting. It is more common in men. In Britain, about 1 man in 10 will suffer angina at some time. Men with diabetes and men from the Indian subcontinent are more liable than others to suffer angina.

Angina is a symptom of the very common artery disease atherosclerosis which affects many arteries in the body, causing narrowing and partial obstruction to the blood flow. In this case, the arteries concerned are the coronary arteries of the heart. These arteries and their branches supply the heart muscle with the oxygen and fuel it needs to keep beating.

If these arteries can provide enough blood so that the heart gets the amount of fuel and oxygen it needs for its energy supply under conditions of exertion, the heart goes on beating painlessly. If the coronary arteries have been narrowed and can't get the blood to the heart muscle fast enough to meet the demand, abnormal levels of substances such as lactic acid collect in the muscle to the point of causing angina .

Symptoms

1 The pain usually comes on after a fixed amount of exertion for each man, such as walking a particular distance.
2 It may be of very variable severity, even in the same person, and may be affected by factors such as cold weather, a change of temperature as when going outside from a warm house, the strength of the wind, the state of your mind, and the length of time since your last meal.
3 The pain can vary enormously. It may be so mild as to be hardly a pain – more a feeling of uneasiness or pressure in the chest – or so severe as to stop you in your tracks.
4 It is often linked with breathlessness and belching but anti-indigestion treatments seldom help.
5 When the exertion ceases, the angina soon settles. It is quite common for angina to remain at a fairly constant level of severity for years.
6 Unstable angina is a severe and dangerous form of angina. Pain becomes more frequent and prolonged, and may occur at rest.
7 With unstable angina it becomes difficult to predict how much exercise will cause pain, and the risk of a heart attack is increased.

Causes

8 Healthy coronary arteries can pass enough blood to allow the heart to reach its maximum output without pain. But narrowing of the coronary arteries will always mean that there is a limit to the rate blood can get to the heart muscle.

9 When a coronary artery, or a branch is reduced in capacity by more than 50% any rise in demand often cannot be fully met.

10 A similar pain can be experienced elsewhere in the body under conditions of inadequate blood supply. If the main artery to the leg, for instance, is narrowed by atherosclerosis, pain occurs in the calf after walking a certain distance (claudication).

Diagnosis

11 An ECG (electrocardiogram), taken during exercise, shows a characteristic pattern. Angina must be distinguished from the pain of a heart attack which often radiates up into the jaw, through to the back and down the left arm. It is associated with severe restlessness and distress and there will seldom be any doubt that something serious has happened.

12 The main difference between this pain and the pain of angina is the length of time it lasts. Generally speaking, angina ceases when you stop doing what brought it on. This can be the important difference between angina and a heart attack which usually lasts for hours and is not relieved by stopping any form of exercise.

13 Thankfully most cases of chest pain are due neither to angina nor to heart attack. Chest pain, however, should always be reported to your doctor. Unless the cause is obvious, it is not a symptom which can safely be ignored.

Prevention

14 Once angina has been diagnosed it can be prevented by keeping within your exertional limits. But that's a bit like closing the stable door after the horse has bolted. Far better to prevent angina earlier in life by healthy living. This is going to be a mantra throughout this book, and no-one ever said it was easy, but trying to avoid cigarette smoking, getting plenty of exercise and a good diet are the most important tips from our experts. In the case of angina, please

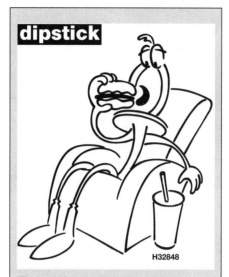

For optimum performance keep your fuel injectors clear of debris

don't try to 'walk through your pain barrier' as advised by less knowledgeable but well meaning people.

Treatment

15 The drug glyceryl trinitrate (nitroglycerine) is highly effective in controlling the pain of angina. The oral preparation may be taken in a tablet that is allowed to dissolve under the tongue and the pain is usually relieved in two to three minutes. The drug is also available in patches to be applied to the skin (transdermal patches) and sprays for under the tongue.

16 Glyceryl trinitrate should not be taken in combination with some other drugs. Ask your GP if you are unsure.

17 An effective treatment for angina is to have your narrowed coronary arteries widened by a procedure called coronary angioplasty.

18 A sausage-shaped balloon segment near one end of a very narrow tube is pushed into the narrowed part of the artery. The balloon is then inflated to widen the constriction before being removed.

19 The alternative to angioplasty, coronary artery bypass, now carries very little risk and the results are excellent. Segments of vein are used to provide a new channel by which the blood can be shunted past the blocked part of the artery.

20 Many surgeons prefer to connect a local artery from the chest wall, a mammary artery, to the narrowed coronary beyond the point of the block.

Action

21 If you have chest pain on exertion, make an appointment to see your GP about it.

2 Atrial fibrillation (irregular heartbeat)

Introduction

The heart has its own natural pacemaker called the sinoatrial node. Its impulses are conveyed from there to another node at the junction between the upper and the lower chambers, called the atrioventricular node.

It is the atrioventricular node that determines the rate of contraction of the lower chambers, the ventricles, and thus the pulse rate.

Atrial fibrillation is a condition in which the upper chambers of the heart

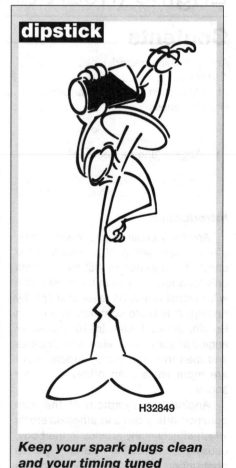

Keep your spark plugs clean and your timing tuned

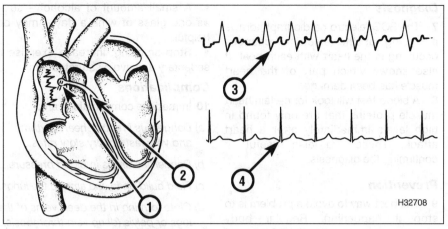

2.3 ECG trace showing atrial fibrillation

1 Sino-atrial node   2 AV node   3 Irregular heart beat   4 Normal heart beat

contracts at a very high rate and in an erratic manner. The result is an irregular beating of the ventricles, which is felt as a 'fluttering' in the chest.

The number of cases of atrial fibrillation in a population increases with age. People who already have heart disease are particularly vulnerable.

Symptoms

1 A 'fluttering' sensation in the chest is the commonest description. Atrial fibrillation is a completely irregular, but usually fast, heart beat rate. It is often in excess of 140 beats per minute, but the rate may be anywhere between 50-200 beats per minute. In the early stages, symptoms seem more prominent.

Causes

2 Overactivity of the thyroid gland, excessive alcohol intake or inflammation of the heart muscle are all common causes

Diagnosis

3 Electrocardiograph (ECG) is vital.
4 Blood tests can also be useful in the diagnosis. They may show anaemia, which may be complicating the situation, impaired kidney function, thyroid gland over activity (thyrotoxicosis).

Prevention

5 Regular checks on blood pressure and treatment for raised pressure can reduce the chances of developing the heart problems that cause atrial fibrillation.

Complications

6 The risk of stroke in people with atrial fibrillation is about twice that in the general population.

Treatment

7 The first step is to be sure whether the cause of the atrial fibrillation is known and can be treated. If so, this may be all the treatment that is required.
8 Digoxin is a well established way of controlling atrial fibrillation, but beta blockers or the calcium channel blockers, or a combination of these drugs, can also help.
9 Cardioversion (electric shock to the heart under general anaesthetic) is most likely to be successful.

Action

10 Make an appointment to see your GP.

---

3   Heart attack

Introduction

An acute myocardial infarction (heart attack) is what happens when the blood supply to a part of the heart muscle has been cut off by blockage of one of the coronary arteries.

When blood is restricted or cut off the cells start to die.

Heart attack is the final result of a disease of the heart arteries (coronary artery disease) called atherosclerosis. About five people in every 1000, mostly

men, suffer a heart attack in the UK each year.

Symptoms

1 A heart attack can involve:
a) *Crushing central chest pain (often described as a 'vice around the chest').*
b) *Breathlessness.*
c) *Clammy skin, sweating and pale complexion.*
d) *Dizziness, nausea and vomiting.*
e) *Restlessness.*
2 The pain often travels to the neck, jaws, ears, arms and wrists. Less often, it travels to between the shoulder blades or to the stomach. The pain does not pass on resting as in angina (see angina).
3 Severe pain is not always present. In less major cases pain may be absent and there is evidence that up to 20% of mild heart attacks are not recognised as such, or even as significant illness, by those affected.

Causes

4 Blockage of the coronary arteries

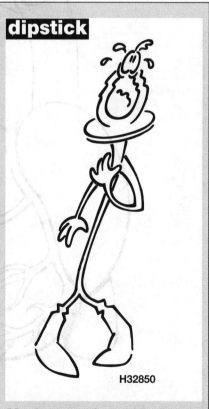

dipstick

H32850

Much worse than a blockage on the M25

3

caused by a clot (thrombosis) from fatty material caught in the blood.

5 When total blockage occurs, part of the heart muscle loses its blood supply and dies. Depending on the size of the artery blocked, a larger or smaller portion of the heart will be affected.

6 Risk factors include:

a) *Smoking cigarettes.*

b) *Being overweight.*

c) *Abnormally high blood pressure.*

d) *High blood cholesterol level.*

e) *A diet high in saturated fats (animal fats).*

f) *Diabetes.*

g) *A family history of heart disease.*

h) *Lack of regular exercise.*

Diagnosis

7 The ECG (electro cardiograph) draws a tracing of the electrical changes occurring in the heart with each beat. It also shows which part of the heart muscle has been damaged.

8 A blood test will look for certain heart muscle proteins that are only found in high levels immediately after a heart attack. These are also useful in confirming the diagnosis.

Prevention

9 The best way to avoid a problem is to stop it happening. Regular body maintenance using the right fuels and getting regular run-outs will help. Here are some pointers:

• Your diet should include a high proportion of fruit and fresh vegetables.

• A small amount of alcohol – such as one glass of wine a day – may be helpful.

• Stop smoking, increase exercise if sedentary and avoid saturated fats.

Complications

10 Immediate complications are:

a) *Dangerous irregular heart rhythms and very fast or very slow rates.*

b) *Dangerous drops in blood pressure.*

c) *Fluid build-up in and around the lungs.*

d) *Clots forming in the deep veins of the legs or pelvis (deep vein thrombosis).*

e) *Rupture of the heart wall.*

11 Later complications are:

a) *Ballooning (aneurysm) of the damaged heart wall, which becomes thin and weak.*

b) *Increased risk of another heart attack in the future.*

c) *Angina.*

d) *Poor heart action causing breathlessness and build-up of fluid in the ankles and legs (oedema).*

e) *Depression, loss of confidence, loss of sex drive, and fear of having sex which is common and unfounded.*

Treatment

12 See Cardio-Pulmonary Resuscitation (Kiss of Life) in Chapter 1.

13 Clot-dissolving injections are now routinely used in hospital. These can break down the clot in the coronary artery and allow the damaged heart muscle to recover, sometimes completely. They must be given within 24 hours at the most. Because the heart rhythm may become temporarily abnormal as it recovers, this treatment is best given when the heart rhythm can be continuously monitored on an ECG. This can be done in an ambulance or in hospital.

14 In an uncomplicated recovery it is normal to be home within a week or less. Work can be restarted 4–12 weeks after the attack, depending on the level of physical exertion involved with the job. Driving can restart after one month, but DVLA and the motor insurance company must be informed of the heart attack.

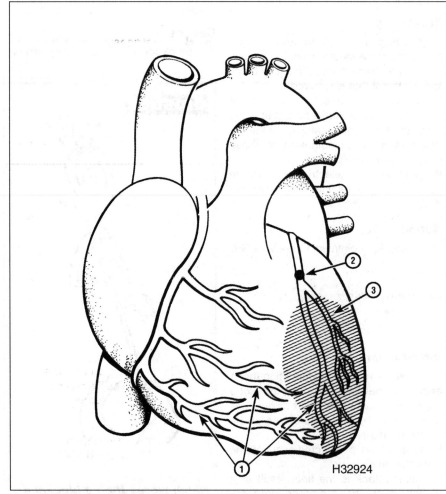

3.1 Heart and blood vessels showing what happens in a heart attack

1 Coronary arteries   2 Blockage   3 Oxygen starved tissue

H32924

15 Rather than avoiding any exercise it is now known that a return to normal levels of activity – this includes sex – helps prevent any further attacks.

4 Heart failure

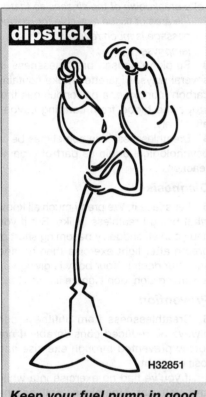

dipstick

H32851

Keep your fuel pump in good working order to make sure of an even flow

Introduction

A frightening term but heart failure actually means that the heart is not pumping quite as efficiently as it could, not that the whole thing has collapsed.
Heart failure can be treated once it is recognised.

Symptoms

1 Breathlessness, particularly when lying down flat is the most distressing symptom (many people find a couple of pillows helps). A wheezing or bubbling noise may sometimes be heard which clears on sitting up.
2 Breathlessness can also happen during mild activity such as climbing stairs.
3 Fluid may build up in the ankles causing swelling. This will be most noticeable in the evening after a day of walking or sitting.

Causes

4 A number of things can cause the heart not to work efficiently. Leaking heart valves from an infection like rheumatic fever or a previous heart attack are among the most common causes. Sometimes this affects one side of the heart more than the other and the symptoms can be slightly different, but breathlessness is often the result.

Prevention

5 There are lots of ways of reducing your risk from heart disease. If you haven't already, go back and read the expert tips on diet and exercise in routine maintenance. Your body will only function with the right fuel and then being thoroughly run in.

Complications

6 Lack of treatment may cause the heart to become further weakened making the breathlessness even worse.

Self care

7 There is no good reason for avoiding exercise and keeping active is important so long as it doesn't put too much strain on the heart.
8 Swollen ankles will benefit from putting your feet up while sitting down.
9 Cut down on your salt and/or use salt substitutes.

Treatment

10 Modern medicines make an enormous difference not only to the quality of life but also life expectancy.

Action

11 If you think you are suffering from heart failure from the symptoms described, call NHS Direct, your GP or dial 999/112 in an emergency.
12 A severe onset of breathlessness, particularly in a person with previously diagnosed heart failure, is a medical emergency – dial 999/112.

5 Breathlessness

Introduction

Being breathless is a normal part of everyday life and for lots of different

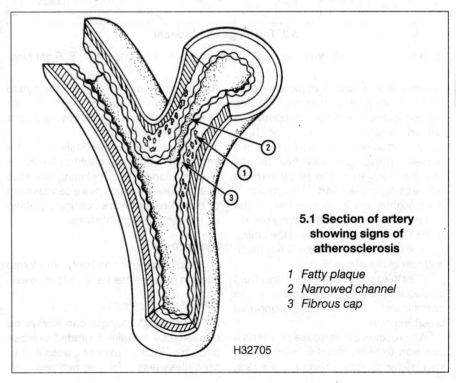

5.1 Section of artery showing signs of atherosclerosis

1 Fatty plaque
2 Narrowed channel
3 Fibrous cap

H32705

3

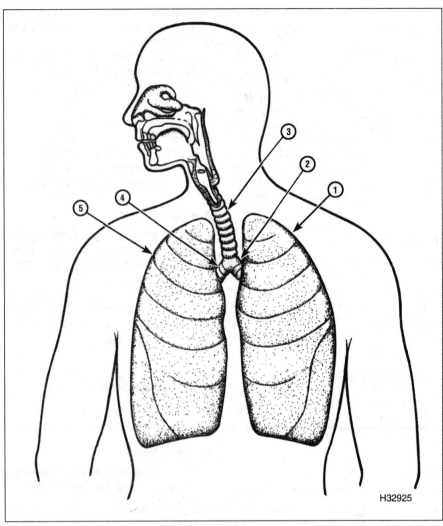

5.2 The lungs and bronchi

1 Left lung   2 Left bronchus   3 Trachea   4 Right bronchus   5 Right lung

reasons. It is a natural response to the bodily system that detects that the oxygen in the blood has dropped. The carotid arteries in the neck have small clumps of cells called the carotid bodies. These are sensitive to the levels of oxygen in the blood passing upwards from the heart. If this blood is even slightly low in oxygen the carotid bodies will send messages, along nerves, to the vital breathing centres in the brain.

The result is an increase in the depth and rate of breathing.

Breathlessness from unfitness from inadequate exercise is probably the commonest form of abnormal breathlessness.

Atherosclerosis (disease of arteries) can lead to heart attacks, heart failure, strokes and other severe disorders.

Almost any heart disorder can cause abnormal breathlessness, so atherosclerosis is, indirectly, a major cause of breathlessness.

People who are seriously unfit at a time in life when they ought to be fit, are in some danger of developing diseases that will cause a much more serious form of breathlessness than ordinary puffing on the second flight of stairs.

Symptoms

1 Breathlessness on only moderate exertion means either being unfit or unwell.

Causes

2 Unfit breathlessness can always be corrected by sustained, graded exercise and by losing excess weight but breathlessness is sometimes an important sign of disease. Conditions that will always cause breathlessness for this reason include:

a) *asthma.*

b) *lung collapse due to air leaking between the lung and the chest wall (pneumothorax).*

c) *acute bronchitis.*

d) *chronic bronchitis.*

e) *a breakdown of the air sacs so that the area of tissue available for oxygen passage is much reduced (emphysema).*

3 Smoking causes breathlessness in several ways. Cigarette smoke contains carbon monoxide, a poisonous gas that stops the blood from carrying oxygen effectively.

4 Breathlessness can sometimes be of psychological origin as part of a panic reaction.

Diagnosis

5 Let's face it. We pretty much all know what being breathless is like. But if you find yourself suddenly becoming short of breath after light exercise then go and see your doctor. Your body is giving you a warning sign, don't ignore it.

Prevention

6 Breathlessness from unfitness can always be reduced considerably if not totally prevented through exercise and losing weight.

7 If you've had no exercise in a while and you get breathless, pull on the trainers and give the man machine a good run. Start with some light exercise and work up. The British Heart Foundation can offer help and advice on getting and staying fitter.

Treatment

8 The cause of the breathlessness needs to be diagnosed and treated.

Action

9 Abnormal breathlessness should not be ignored. Make an appointment to see your GP

Further information

10 If you would like to know more, look in the Contacts section at the back of this manual, or contact:

British Heart Foundation,
14 Fitzhardinge Street,
London, W1H 6DH.
020 7935 0185
www.bhf.org.uk

6 Asthma

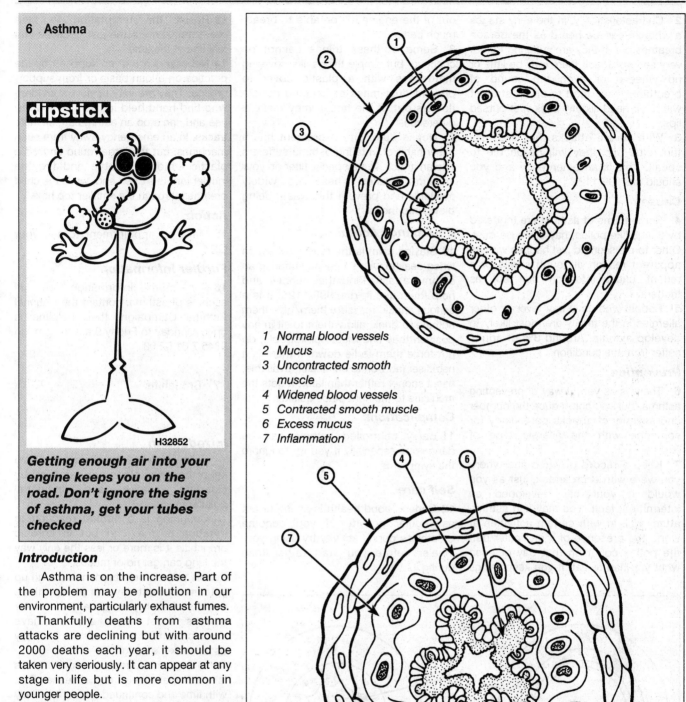

dipstick

H32852

Getting enough air into your engine keeps you on the road. Don't ignore the signs of asthma, get your tubes checked

1 Normal blood vessels
2 Mucus
3 Uncontracted smooth muscle
4 Widened blood vessels
5 Contracted smooth muscle
6 Excess mucus
7 Inflammation

H32710

6.1 Normal (top) and asthmatic airways

Introduction

Asthma is on the increase. Part of the problem may be pollution in our environment, particularly exhaust fumes.

Thankfully deaths from asthma attacks are declining but with around 2000 deaths each year, it should be taken very seriously. It can appear at any stage in life but is more common in younger people.

Some people find the severity of the condition decreases as they get older. Thankfully modern treatments will prevent or stop the vast majority of asthma attacks.

Symptoms

1 The first sign of an attack can be as simple as a persistent cough which can rapidly develop into a frightening breathlessness and tightness in the chest.

2 Characteristically, in the early stages a wheeze can be heard as the person breathes out. If they are suffering from a very serious attack there may be little or no wheeze or even the sound of breathing. They tend to sit up straight with their head slightly back with pursed lips.

3 With severe attacks their lips may turn blue and they will be unable to speak. This is an emergency and you should dial 999/112.

Causes

4 Some forms of asthma are triggered by things like pollen, hay or house dust. Other forms seem to just happen with no apparent reason although stress or a recent chest infection can act as triggers.

5 People who have hay fever or other allergies in the family are most likely to develop asthma. Around 3% of adults suffer from the condition.

Prevention

6 There is as yet no way of preventing asthma, but you can reduce the number and severity of attacks particularly for someone with the allergic type of asthma.

7 Keep a record of when and where you were with each attack, just as you would if your car developed an intermittent fault. You may find asthma attacks tie in with certain activities at work, the presence of a particular pet, the pollen count on that day or even what you had to eat. If you keep things

out of the engine it'll be able to breath much better.

8 Some of these things cannot be changed, but simple things like covering mattresses with a plastic cover to prevent dust mites or keeping certain flowers out of the house may make a difference.

9 House dust mite excrement has a nasty habit of irritating asthma sufferers into an attack. Put a special filter on your vacuum cleaner. These are widely available and prevent this waste being blown into the air.

Emergency Action

10 Staying calm is the most vital action when dealing with someone suffering an asthma attack. Find their inhaler and help them use it, dial 999/112 if it is a serious attack, reassure them, give them nothing to drink, allow them to sit in any position they find most comfortable, do not force them to lie down. If there is a nebuliser (add-on to an inhaler) available, use it sooner rather than later. It gets the medicine to the right place quicker.

Complications

11 Badly controlled asthma can be dangerous especially if you try to ignore the symptoms.

Self care

12 General good health is as important as regular activity. If you become breathless during activity try using your inhaler before you start rather than during it.

13 Resist the temptation to skip preventative medicine just because you feel fine at the time.

14 Nebulisers are often supplied by the practice on a loan basis or from support groups. They are very useful for children who find hand held inhalers difficult to use and can stop an asthma attack in its tracks. In an emergency away from such machines, cut the large round end off a plastic lemonade bottle and fire the inhaler into this open end, while the child breathes through the smaller top hole.

Action

15 Make an appointment to see your GP.

Further information

16 For more information on all aspects of asthma, contact the National Asthma Campaign, their helpline is open Monday to Friday 9 am to 7pm, on 0845 7 01 02 03.

7 Bronchitis

Introduction

Cells which line the airways and help keep the lungs clean are damaged by cigarette smoke and industrial pollutants.

Coughing is a natural reaction to irritation of the lung but in chronic bronchitis it is more or less the only way the lung can get rid of mucus.

People with chronic bronchitis cough up sputum on most days for at least three months of each year, usually the winter months. Most heavy smokers have chronic bronchitis, but refer to it simply as 'a smoker's cough'.

In the early stages, chronic bronchitis is a comparatively mild disease. But, with time and continued abuse, it is likely to progress to the condition called chronic obstructive airway disease (COAD), chronic obstructive pulmonary disease (COPD) or emphysema. Large numbers of the tiny lung air sacs break down to form a smaller number of larger air spaces.

Smoking is especially dangerous in people with a persistent, productive cough. Chronic bronchitis and other forms of COAD / COPD affect 18% of male smokers.

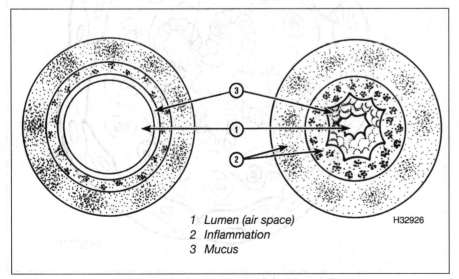

1 Lumen (air space)
2 Inflammation
3 Mucus

H32926

7.1 Normal (left) and inflamed bronchi

Symptoms

1 In acute bronchitis there is a cough, at first dry but later with sputum, maybe fever for a few days, breathlessness and wheezing. There may be some pain in the chest. Occasionally a little blood may be coughed up.

Causes

2 Acute bronchitis in a previously healthy person is usually due to infection with a virus. In cigarette smokers this is often followed by additional infection by other germs that makes matters worse. Industrial atmospheric pollution may also be a cause.

3 Most experts are convinced that by far the most important factor in the causation of serious bronchitis is cigarette smoking.

Diagnosis

4 Bronchitis causes characteristic sounds audible to a health professional on listening with a stethoscope.

5 In peak expiratory flow measurement in a normal person, asked to breathe out as forcibly as possible through the mouth, the rate of flow of the air rises rapidly to a peak and then declines steadily to zero. A normal person can breathe out at a peak rate of up to 8 litres a second, but in certain lung diseases, such as bronchitis, because of narrowing or partial obstruction of the bronchial tubes, the figure is much lower.

Prevention

6 You don't need an expert to work out the best way to prevent chronic bronchitis. Quit smoking, lay off the tabs, kick the wicked weed. See the routine maintenance section on stopping smoking. However, you might need some expert advice on the best way to give up.

Complications

7 The increased resistance to blood passing through the lungs imposes an additional load on the heart which responds by enlarging. Up to a point, the increased power of the enlarged ventricle enables the heart to compensate, but eventually the heart muscle fails and the blood returning to it from the rest of the body cannot be pumped fast enough.

Treatment

8 Acute bronchitis is often treated with antibiotics and usually responds well, although it may be necessary to use oxygen in severe cases. There is no cure for chronic bronchitis, but not smoking can do much to improve it. Various other drugs can help.

Action

9 Make an appointment to see your GP.

Further information

10 Contact Quit for more information and practical support:

QUIT,
Ground Floor,
211 Old Street,
London,
EC1V 9NR.
Smokers' Quit-line: 0800 00 22 00
www.quit.org.uk

8 Lung cancer

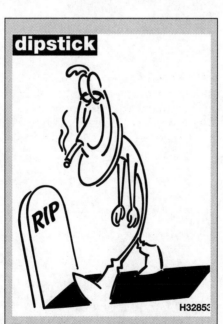

Don't end up an insurance write-off. Give up the cigs

Introduction

Cancer of the large tubes of the lung is called bronchial carcinoma, 'lung cancer'. The lining cells of the air tubes in healthy lungs are tall and the surfaces nearest the inside of the tube are covered with fine hairs (cilia) which move together.

The movement of the cilia acts to carry dust and smoke particles and other foreign material upwards and away from the deeper parts of the lungs. Smoking cigarettes causes important changes not least on the cilia which disappear and the cells become flattened, so that they are replaced by an abnormal, scaly layer. Some years later it may develop into lung cancer.

Lung cancer is uncommon before the age of 40. Only about 1 case in 100 is diagnosed in people younger than 40. The great majority of cases (85%) occur in people over 60.

After diagnosis of the disease life expectancy for most men is one year. Only 8%, overall, survive for five years.

Symptoms

1 Lung cancer usually shows itself with a productive cough and there is often a little blood in the sputum. There may also be breathlessness. Pain in the chest is common, especially if the cancer has spread to the lung lining (pleura) or the chest wall.

2 Unfortunately the tumour may show no signs until late in its development.

Causes

3 It is mostly due to cigarette smoking.

4 Passive smoking is another known cause. The rate of lung cancer in non-smokers rises significantly if they are regularly exposed to other people's cigarette smoke.

Diagnosis

5 X-ray examination usually shows a suspicious shadow.

6 Sometimes the diagnosis can only be made by examining the inside of the bronchi with a bronchoscope (telescopic camera). If a tumour is seen, a sample (biopsy) is usually taken for examination. Cancer cells can sometimes be found in the sputum.

Prevention

7 Stop smoking. Full stop.

Action

8 Make an appointment to see your GP.

3

Notes

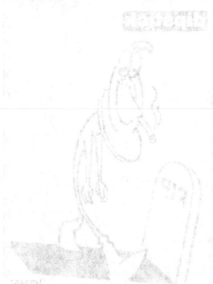

Chapter 4
Cooling systems (circulation)

Contents

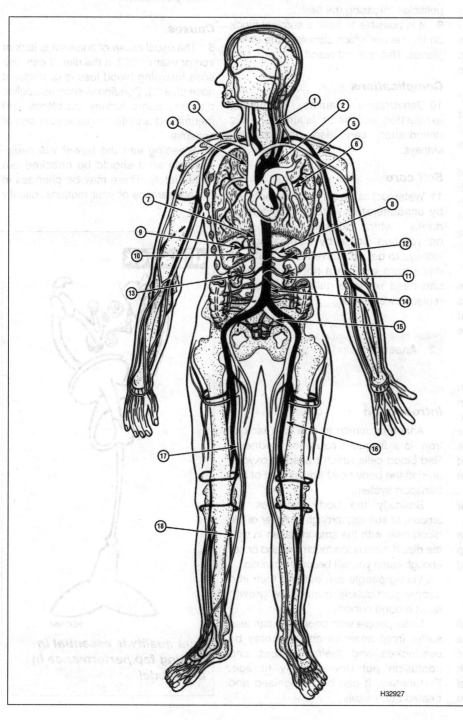

The major blood vessels

1 Carotid artery
2 Ascending aorta
3 Subclavian vein
4 Superior vena cava
5 Subclavian artery
6 Pulmonary artery
7 Inferior vena cava
8 Splenic artery
9 Hepatic artery
10 Hepatic vein
11 Renal vein
12 Splenic vein
13 Renal artery
14 Abdominal aorta
15 Common iliac vein
16 Femoral artery
17 Femoral vein
18 Great saphenous vein

H32927

4

1 Sweat

Introduction

1 Sweat is a mixture of water, salts and a little protein. It is produced by the skin's sweat glands which are found all over the body but tend to be more concentrated in areas like the hands. Although the skin is a major detoxifying organ the production of sweat is mainly part of temperature control. The evaporation of the water has a dramatic cooling effect, especially if there is free movement of air over the skin.

2 Clothes act as 'double glazing' trapping air heated by the body. Sweat evaporation is also prevented which is why totally impervious material like plastic produces dampness.

3 We can lose very large amounts of body water by sweating in high temperatures or during a fever which must be replaced as the body cannot withstand dehydration for more than a day or so.

Symptoms

4 Profuse sweating can be embarrassing but rarely dangerous unless there is also significant dehydration. Lack of sweating can cause overheating.

Causes

5 The main cause is a high environmental temperature but it can also occur with a fever. It is important to reduce the amount of clothes to allow this sweat to evaporate and cool the body as the brain in particular cannot tolerate high temperatures. A fan can help cool someone that much quicker.

6 Inappropriate sweating can occur from alcohol abuse and anxiety.

7 The smell of under-arm sweat comes from bacteria which like warm damp environments, not from the sweat itself which has little or no smell.

Prevention

8 Right, no sweat. That really is a tall order for our tradesmen. It might be embarrassing, always happening at the worst times, but sweating is vital. Fresh sweat should have no smell, so the most important tip is to wash regularly to prevent stale sweat. Sparing use of antiperspirants will help, but many so-called deodorants simply mask the smell and do not stop sweating. Dress appropriately for the weather and lose excess weight, it'll stop your body working so hard and having to get rid of excess heat. Rinsing sweaty hands in a dilute solution of aluminium chloride (from your pharmacist) will stop sweating for many hours, useful if you are a politician 'pressing the flesh'.

9 It is possible to have a surgical block on the nerves which stimulate the sweat glands. This is a last resort.

Complications

10 Dehydration causes confusion, exhaustion and heart failure. Chronic dehydration can also damage the kidneys.

Self care

11 Water lost as sweat must be replaced by unadulterated water, not alcoholic drinks which simply make the dehydration worse by stimulating the kidneys to get rid of even more water. A day's hard work in a hot environment can need up to a gallon of water to replace sweat alone.

2 Anaemia

Introduction

Anaemia, which is due to a lack of iron, is a frequent cause of tiredness. Red blood cells which transport oxygen around the body need iron as part of this transport system.

Basically the body balances the amount of iron lost through turnover of the blood cells with the amount taken in with the diet. If there is too much lost and or not enough eaten you will become anaemic.

Young people can outstrip their iron supply particularly during the growth spurt around puberty.

Older people with poor diets can also suffer from anaemia and this may be overlooked and their tiredness and confusion put down simply to age. Fortunately, it can be recognised and treated quite easily

Symptoms

1 Skin, lips, tongue, nail beds or the inside of eyelids can be pale in colour although this doesn't really happen until your iron stores are quite low.

2 Tiredness and weakness.

3 Dizziness or fainting spells.

4 Breathlessness, particularly following exercise.

5 Fast heartbeat felt in the neck or chest (palpitations).

Causes

6 The usual cause of anaemia is lack of iron or vitamin B12 in the diet. It can also arise following blood loss (e.g. frequent nose bleeds). Conditions such as coeliac disease, some kidney problems and rheumatoid arthritis increase your risk of anaemia.

7 Bleeding into the bowel will cause anaemia so it should be checked out immediately. There may be changes in the appearance of your motions, usually

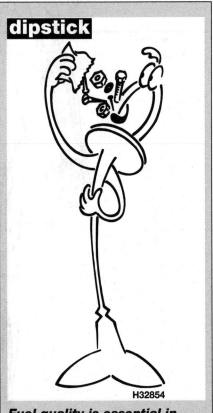

Fuel quality is essential in getting top performance in any model

a black tar like substance and you may lose weight for no apparent reason.

Prevention

8 Being anaemic is not just about looking slightly pasty faced. Our tip for tip-top blood is to eat a balanced diet to supply all the minerals you need. Young boys going through their growth spurt need to make sure they are eating enough bread and other iron containing foods.

9 Meat is a major source of iron which is great news for carnivores, but if you are a vegetarian, you'll need extra iron containing foods – spinach and dark green veg is good – and may even benefit from iron supplements.

Complications

10 Anaemia itself is not usually life threatening but it can cause accidents through tiredness and lower your defence against minor illness.

Treatment

11 If you suspect you are anaemic and there is no obvious reason for being so do

not start iron supplements until you have had blood tests performed and your doctor has advised you. Taking iron before the test makes it difficult to tell why you became anaemic in the first place.

12 If anaemia is confirmed by a blood test, your doctor may prescribe iron tablets or injections or, occasionally, vitamin B12 injections. You can also help yourself by eating plenty of iron-rich foods, such as red meat, wholemeal bread, dried fruit and leafy vegetables.

Action

13 Make an appointment to see your GP.

3 Erectile dysfunction (impotence)

Introduction

Problems with erections are common. More than half of all men over 40 report some form of erectile

dysfunction (ED) at some stage of their lives. ED is not the same as infertility. A man can father children without being able to have an erection.

Misery on this scale is often masked by men's understandable reluctance to discuss these problems, despite the fact that many of them can be overcome by relatively simple treatments. This reluctance also covers up other problems such as breakdown in relationships, and depression amongst men with ED.

For most cases of ED there will be a varying mixture of psychological and physical causes, along with adverse affects of medicines. Around 20 to 30% of all cases will be purely psychological (resulting from stress or anxiety) and will often respond well to non-clinical treatments such as sex counselling.

Generally speaking, if you have erections at any time other than during attempted intercourse then you are more likely to have a psychological rather than physical problem. Successful erections during television programmes, sexy

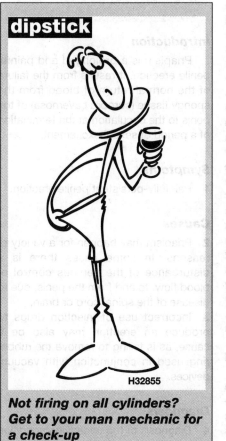

dipstick

Not firing on all cylinders?
Get to your man mechanic for
a check-up

H32855

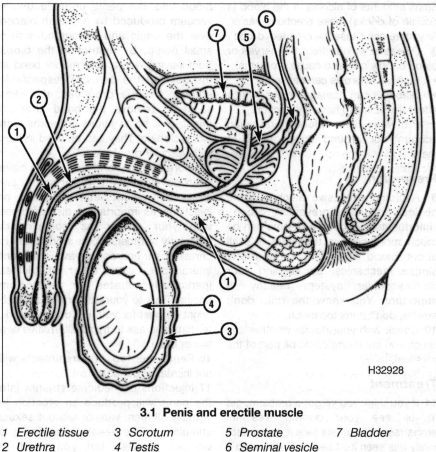

3.1 Penis and erectile muscle

1 *Erectile tissue*	3 *Scrotum*	5 *Prostate*	7 *Bladder*
2 *Urethra*	4 *Testis*	6 *Seminal vesicle*	

H32928

videos or masturbation bodes well for the future, although it is not a 100% test.

Symptoms

1 Being unable to establish and / or maintain an erection sufficient for making love is about the best description.
2 ED usually has a gradual onset.

Causes

3 The penis works by hydrostatic pressure from allowing blood in to the spongy tissues of the penis but restricting its outflow.
4 Anything which affects the arteries, veins or nerves which bring this about will influence the ability to have an erection.
5 Some medicines cause problems with erections, so talk to your doctor if you are worried.
6 Certain anti depressives can make ED worse and some blood pressure drugs are common culprits.
7 Alcohol is a common cause. Obviously binge drinking has an immediate effect but chronic alcohol abuse can lead to permanent problems. Small amounts of alcohol in the blood (a couple of drinks) make erections easier. Any more can cause the dreaded 'droop'.
8 Diseases which affect the nerves or blood supply can also cause problems:
• Multiple sclerosis can cause ED.
• Diabetes can damage nerves, which affect the ability to have an erection.
• Problems with blood circulation account for around 25% of ED in men.

Prevention

9 Avoiding excessive alcohol is the obvious first line to preventing 'droop'. Unfortunately erection problems can be much more serious than that. It's all about blood flow, and some pretty simple mechanics, so keeping your cardiovascular system healthy is important. You know the drill, don't smoke, don't drink too much.
10 Check with your doctor whether any drugs you are taking could be part of the problem.

Treatment

11 If you think you've got a problem, get in to see your doctor. Yes its embarrassing, but lets face it, the doctor really has seen it all before. Try to keep it business-like to prevent embarrassment. Bring along a checklist of questions to ask, and think about answers to these common questions ready:
• Are you currently drinking heavily or finding yourself under heavy stress?
• When was the last time you successfully had sexual intercourse?
• Do you wake up with an erection (so called 'morning glory')?
12 However, it's not just about the doctor asking you questions. ED can seriously affect who you are. So think about how different treatments might affect your normal sex life.
13 Remember that in the majority of cases ED can be effectively treated, and by working with your GP you will get the best treatment. Your doctor is no mind reader, so if he gives you a treatment and it doesn't work (give it some time though, some treatments need a few goes for best results), you are quite within your rights to go back and tell him. There may be other treatments that can be tried.
14 Vacuum devices have been around for over 70 years. They work by drawing blood into the penis under a gentle vacuum produced by a sheath placed over the penis and evacuated with a small pump. By restricting the blood from leaving with a tight rubber band at the base of the penis, a respectable erection can be produced. It makes sense to remove the band after 30 minutes or so to avoid problems with blood clotting. They can be used in men with vascular problems.
15 More recently oral treatments have been developed which, for some, are more convenient than devices or injections. Its important to discuss these with your doctor as some work differently to others; some work better in certain men, and some have important interactions with other medicines (particularly nitrates for relief from angina). Talk to your doctor about which might be best for you. If it doesn't work, tell him, and ask to try an alternative or a higher dose.
16 Remember too, oral treatments will not increase your sex drive.
17 Injections of medicine straight into the penis will produce an erection in virtually all men, with or without sexual stimulation. The needle is so fine it is virtually painless but you need to inject into different places to stop any scarring.
18 Herbal and traditional remedies are freely available but there is little evidence that they work. Most contain yohimbine, a bark extract which at best can only be described as marginally useful.

Further Information

19 For more idea of what your doctor will ask, contact the Impotence Association, their helpline is confidential and will give you lots of practical advice.

Impotence Association,
(For information and advice on all sexual dysfunctions)
PO Box 10296,
London,
SW17 9WH.
020 8767 7791
www.impotence.org.uk

4 Prolonged erections (priapism)

Introduction

Priapism is a prolonged and painful penile erection. It results from the failure of the normal return of blood from the spongy tissue (corpora cavernosa) of the penis to the circulation at the termination of a period of sexual excitement.

Symptoms

1 Painfully-persistent penile erection.

Causes

2 Priapism may happen for a variety of reasons. In some cases there is a disturbance of the nervous control of blood flow, to and from the penis, due to disease of the spinal cord or brain.
3 Incorrect use of injection drugs to produce an erection may also be a cause, as is failing to remove the rubber ring used in conjunction with vacuum devices.

Diagnosis

4 Diagnosis of the underlying condition is important.

Complications

5 A long sustained erection is dangerous because of the risk of a blood clot in the penis, which may produce severe and permanent loss of erectile function, so treatment must be prompt and effective.

Treatment

6 It is possible to reverse the effects of drugs used for producing erections by injecting the penis with other drugs. This may also be useful for other causes of priapism. In rare cases it may be necessary to remove blood from the penis using a syringe.

Action

7 Priapism requires hospital treatment. Go without delay to an accident and emergency department.

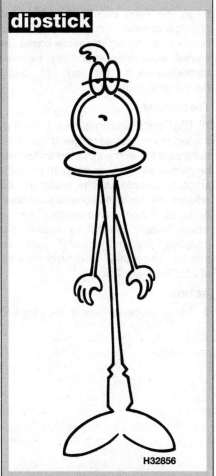

dipstick

The only thing which should remain permanently hard is a gearstick

H32856

5 High blood pressure (hypertension)

Introduction

Myths surround every aspect of blood pressure. It helps to know what is being measured in the first place. Blood pressure (BP) is always written as two numbers thus: 120/80. Neither of these numbers has anything to do with your age, height or weight. They are simple measurements of the heart's ability to overcome pressure from an inflated cuff placed around the arm or leg.

As the cuff is slowly deflated, the sound of the blood pushing its way past is suddenly heard in a stethoscope placed over the artery. This is the maximum pressure reached by the heart during its contraction. As the pressure is further released the sound gradually muffles and disappears. This is the lowest pressure in your blood system. Putting the two pressures over each other gives a ratio of the blood pressure while the heart is contracting (systolic) over the pressure while the heart is refilling with blood ready for the next contraction (diastolic). The lower pressure actually represents the pressure caused by the major arteries contracting, keeping the blood moving while the heart refills.

There is no 'normal' blood pressure as it constantly changes within the same person and depends on what they are doing at the time. A blood pressure above 140/90 for anyone at rest should be investigated.

Symptoms

1 Hypertension is called the silent killer for good reason. Most people do not realise that they are suffering from high

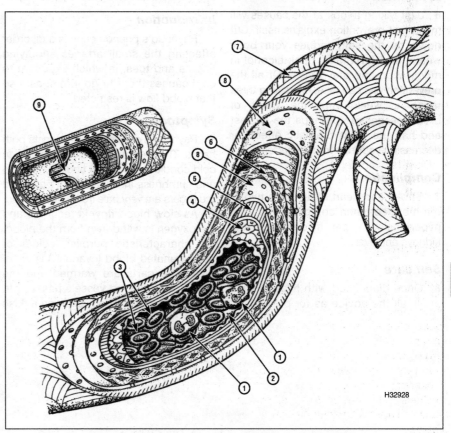

Blood vessel construction - artery (right) and vein

1	*White blood cells*	6	*Tunica media*
2	*Platelets*	7	*Tunica adventitia*
3	*Red blood cells*	8	*Elastic layer*
4	*Tunica intima (inner layer)*	9	*Non-return valve*
5	*Tunica intima (outer layer)*		

H32928

4

blood pressure until something serious happens.

2 As the pressure steadily rises, damage occurs to the arteries, kidney and heart. For this reason alone it is worth having your blood pressure checked every year or so when you are over the age of 45 years.

3 There may be some warning signs such as blood in your urine or loss of vision right at the edges (tunnel vision).

Causes

4 Hypertension can be linked to genetic factors, and this risk is increased by high salt intake, fatty food, obesity, stress, alcohol abuse and lack of activity.

5 Hypertension can also be caused by other medical conditions, which have an effect on blood pressure. Kidney problems are a good example of this.

Prevention

6 Just taking a look at the causes will mean that prevention explains itself. Cut down on the salt, reduce your body weight and fat intake, drink alcohol in moderation and stay active. Of all the prevention you can take, exercising three times a week until the point of breathlessness is perhaps the easiest and has the most dramatic effect for decreasing your risk from hypertension.

Complications

7 Stroke and heart attacks are two of the most common complications from hypertension. It can also damage the kidneys and liver.

Self care

8 Once diagnosed with hypertension apply all the advice as for prevention.

Your doctor may well find that through losing weight, increasing activity and reducing alcohol intake you can do without the medication to bring down your blood pressure.

Note

9 A single reading of blood pressure is unreliable. At least three readings over a few weeks are required. Simply having your blood pressure checked can make it rise in some people (called the white coat effect). Self testing using machines from the pharmacist is a good idea.

Action

10 Make an appointment to see your GP.

6 Raynaud's phenomenon

Introduction

Raynaud's phenomenon is a disorder affecting the small arteries supplying fingers and toes, in which exposure to cold causes them to go into spasm so that blood flow is restricted.

Symptoms

1 Raynaud's disease usually affects both hands. The toes are less often affected. In cold conditions, there is tingling, burning and numbness in the affected parts and the fingers are very pale from lack of blood.

2 As slow blood flow is resumed and the oxygen is withdrawn from the blood, the characteristic purplish colour of deoxygenated blood (cyanosis) is seen. When the parts are warmed and the spasm of the blood vessels passes off, the vessels open widely, allowing a flush of fresh blood to pass. In this stage, the fingers or toes become red.

Causes

3 Raynaud's phenomenon often occurs in men with underlying illnesses affecting the arteries, it sometimes affects those using vibrating power tools or pneumatic drills.

Diagnosis

4 This is based on the characteristic physical signs (colour changes) that occur on exposure to cold.

Prevention

5 People suffering from Raynaud's disease must avoid cold and keep the extremities well insulated. Cigarette smoking is especially dangerous as it increases the constriction of the small arteries.

Complications

6 In the early months or years, no physical change occurs in the affected blood vessels, but in severe cases the vessel walls may eventually become thickened and the flow of blood permanently reduced.

Treatment

7 Raynaud's phenomenon is treated by correcting the cause, if this is possible, but treatment of the symptoms may also be necessary. Various drugs to relax the smooth muscle in the walls of the arteries are useful in Raynaud's disease.

8 Cutting of the sympathetic nerves which supply the blood vessel wall muscles (sympathectomy) can be helpful, especially when the disease affects the lower limb.

Action

9 Make an appointment to see your GP.

Chapter 5
Engine management system (brain)

Contents

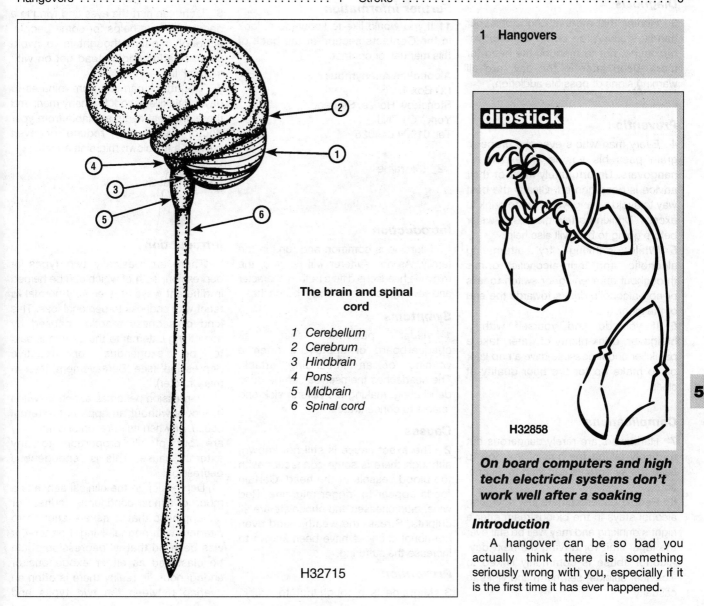

The brain and spinal cord

1 Cerebellum
2 Cerebrum
3 Hindbrain
4 Pons
5 Midbrain
6 Spinal cord

H32715

1 Hangovers

dipstick

H32858

On board computers and high tech electrical systems don't work well after a soaking

Introduction

A hangover can be so bad you actually think there is something seriously wrong with you, especially if it is the first time it has ever happened.

5

Symptoms

1 Headache, nausea, tiredness and thirst are the commonest symptoms.

Causes

2 Dehydration is the main cause. Alcohol acts as a diuretic stimulating the kidneys to lose water. Some alcoholic drinks contain toxins which act as mild poisons. Red wine in excess tends to cause headaches for this reason. Sleep while intoxicated is always poor as the alcohol interferes with the normal sleep pattern. This causes a feeling of not having slept the next morning.

Diagnosis

3 Finding that more alcohol stops your hands shaking or cures a hangover headache, not to mention the need for more sleep later in the day, are all warning signs of possible addiction.

Prevention

4 Every man who's ever had grape or grain pass his lips is an expert on hangovers. Unfortunately most of their advice is best ignored. Clearly the best way to avoid a hangover is not to drink to excess. Drinking a few glasses of water before going to bed will also help.
5 While drinking try alternating alcoholic and non-alcoholic drinks throughout an evening, or switch to less or non-alcoholic drinks towards the end of the night.
6 If you do find yourself with a hangover, drink plenty of water, take a painkiller and if possible have a nap later on to make up for the poor quality of sleep.

Complications

7 Hangovers are rarely dangerous but routinely taking the hair of the dog to ease the symptoms can lead to alcohol abuse.
8 People underestimate just how long alcohol stays in the bloodstream after a night's drinking and may well be still over the legal limit for driving the next day. Alcohol abuse is commonly linked to violence, suicide, self harm and visits to casualty

What service to use

9 See your pharmacist but consider seeing your GP if you feel that alcohol is running your life rather than the other way round.

Action

10 If you are suffering hangovers regularly it is highly likely that you are abusing alcohol and may be becoming dependent on it. If people are commenting on your drinking, you are becoming defensive over it, your work or home relationships are suffering or you are drinking early in the day you should contact support groups such as Alcoholics Anonymous, or contact your GP or pharmacist for advice.

Further information

11 If you would like to know more, look in the Contacts section at the back of this manual, or contact:

Alcoholics Anonymous
PO Box 1
Stonebow House, Stonebow
York YO1 7NJ
Tel: 01904 644026

2 Migraine

Introduction

Migraine is common and runs in the family. As any sufferer will tell you, the migraine headache differs both in character and severity from an 'ordinary' headache.

Symptoms

1 Visual patterns such as chequerboard or spots are often a warning of an impending attack. The headaches themselves can be quite debilitating, making the person sick and unable to concentrate.

Causes

2 The exact cause is still not known, although there is some connection with the blood vessels of the head. Certain foods appear to trigger migraine. Red wine, blue cheeses and chocolate are all culprits. Stress, the weather and even hormonal changes have been known to increase the suffering.

Prevention

3 Migraine is a tough nut to crack.

Avoiding triggers such as red wine or blue cheese seems obvious but different things trigger different people. Try to keep a migraine diary, of both triggers and attacks, and take it with you when you go to the doctor. Our experts agree that your doctor can help. There are loads of treatments so the chances of something working are very high.

Complications

4 The greatest danger from headaches are missing the rare occasion when something more serious is the problem.
5 Your irritability increases and you find you have a greater risk of an accident, as well as abusing painkillers.

Self care

6 Light can hurt the eyes and lying in a darkened room helps for some people, although modern thought is to avoid such isolation and instead get on with 'normal' life.
7 The attack can last from minutes to days. Painkillers work for many men, and there are treatments available from your doctor which may reduce or even prevent a full blown migraine attack.

3 Depression

Introduction

There are basically two types of depression, both of which can be helped in different ways. It is entirely normal to react with sadness to personal loss. This kind of sadness reaction caused by something external to the person is said to be 'exogenous' or 'reactive depression' (see 'Bereavement' later in this Chapter).

Depression becomes abnormal when it occurs without an apparent external cause, or when its duration and intensity are out of all proportion to any external cause. This is 'endogenous depression'.

Depression in the clinical sense is a mood of almost continuous sadness or unhappiness that is severe enough to interfere with normal living. Formerly, it was believed that all depression could be classified as either exogenous or endogenous. In reality there is often an overlap between the two types and

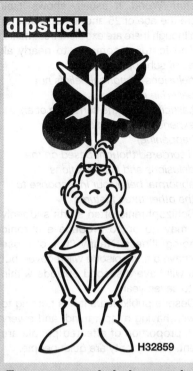

dipstick

H32859

Everyone needs help once in a while. If you're feeling lost don't be afraid to ask for directions

exogenous depression can be every bit as destructive as endogenous.

Clinical depression affects about one person in 100. It is especially common in elderly people. The highest incidence of first attacks occurs between 55 and 65 in men and between 50 and 60 in women.

Depression may run in families but this doesn't necessarily mean that it is wholly genetic in origin.

Symptoms

1 Clinical depression involves a high degree of hopeless despondency, dejection, fear and irritability. Such a degree of sadness in clinical depression is out of all proportion to any external cause. Often there are symptoms such as:
a) *a general slowing down of body and mind.*
b) *insomnia with early morning waking.*
c) *mood worse in the morning.*
d) *slow speech, poor concentration.*
e) *in some cases, restlessness and agitation.*
2 There are also other psychological symptoms, such as:

a) *confusion.*
b) *self-reproach.*
c) *self-accusation.*
d) *loss of self-esteem.*
e) *loss of sexual interest.*
f) *loss of appetite.*

Causes

3 Whilst there are known biochemical changes in the brain associated with depression, it is not clear how these come about. There is a great deal of evidence that by modifying these chemical changes depression can be relieved. The development of antidepressant drugs (see below) has brought this information to light.
4 The seasonal affective disorder syndrome (SADS) is a disorder in which the mood of the affected person changes according to the season of the year. Typically, with the onset of winter, there is depression, general slowing of mind and body, excessive sleeping and overeating. These symptoms resolve with the coming of spring.
5 So far as the causes of reactive depression are concerned, the main causes are bereavement and serious changes in a person's life.

Diagnosis

6 Clinical depression is diagnosed by an interview with the affected person in which it becomes clear that there is a definite mood disorder out of all proportion to any known cause.
7 Don't ever believe that depression is not important. Too many men suffer from what used to be known as the 'black dog', without getting treatment. Despite being the butt of countless jokes, depression isn't funny, you can't just pull yourself together, and depressive men do not just need a good drink.
8 If you see any of yourself, or, just as importantly, your friends in the symptoms above, talk to someone about it. No-one will think you less of a man, and with one in four people suffering from depression in their lifetime, they might surprise you with their insight. Your doctor can help, and the Samaritans provide confidential support.

Treatment

9 Effective antidepressant drugs are available, with complex names such as monoamine oxidase inhibitors, tricyclics, and serotonin re-uptake inhibitors, but the treatment of depression involves more than just prescribing drugs. Skilled investigation of the problem, management and advice can be just as important as drug treatment.
10 For severe cases, electroconvulsive therapy (ECT) is employed, but much less often than formerly, and it may be valuable.

Action

11 Make an appointment to see your GP or ring the Samaritans (08457 90 90 90).

4 Grieving and coping with bereavement

Introduction

Death is inevitably upsetting and may occur at any age, even in childhood. As we grow older, our contact with personal loss increases, but it may never get any easier to deal with.

Death in old age

1 The loss of an elderly relative or friend is supposed to be less painful. People will attempt to console you with well-intended comments such as, 'Well, she had a good innings'. Heads will nod, but a long innings often gives more reason to hope that death will never come.

Scale of misery

2 Psychologists often refer to a scale that rates life events in terms of the stress they can cause. The death of a spouse or child comes at the very top.

Predictable response

3 The scale is useful because it helps to demonstrate how you may feel when you have lost a loved one. The stages of the 'grieving reaction' are listed below. While the order of these stages remains the same for almost everyone, the severity and duration of each will vary from person to person.
a) **Denial:** *'It can't be true. There's been some mistake.'*

5

b) **Anger**: 'It must be the doctor's fault. Why did they leave me?'

c) **Guilt**: The next emotion, self-guilt, can be the most destructive. 'How could I be so idiotic? It's all my fault.' People will find the most unlikely things with which to whip themselves unmercifully. This stage can last a long time even when people rationalise the cause of their misery.

d) **Acceptance**: After a variable amount of time there comes a period of acceptance. There is no fixed time for this period, which can even depend upon the community. People generally will profess to have come to terms with their loss before they have actually done so.

e) **Coming to Terms**: Well-meaning folk will tell you that you'll get over it. The truth is that you never 'get over' a major life event. What happens is that you come to terms with it; the pain diminishes gradually with time. It is not a smooth progression, however, and anniversaries, returning to places, or even casual mention of the person or some object or event will release waves of heartache.

Just to help me sleep

4 People close to the recently bereaved can be so shocked by the effect on their loved one that they may ask for, or even demand, sedatives from the doctor. Your doctor is highly unlikely to give in to these demands. There can be no doubt that drugs will numb the pain of grief. Unfortunately, grief will not be denied; and if it is not allowed to take its course with the support of friends and relatives, it will resurface after the drugs and the support have gone.

5 People in grief then find themselves alone but with the heartache they should have had when help was at hand. People often talk of such an experience as 'floating above the events' only to come down with a thump later on.

Effects underestimated

6 Most people underestimate the effects of bereavement on a person, until it happens to themselves. Some effects can be so bad that the bereaved person often will not realise that loss of interest in job or family, constant pacing of the floor, spontaneous weeping or complete loss of appetite are all normal and common manifestations of grieving.

7 People close to the bereaved person may also become impatient as time wears on, again underestimating the extent of the effects of grief and the length of time they can be felt.

8 It is at this point that true friends are worth their weight in gold. To know when to leave the person alone and when to sit and listen, often to the same story over and over again without interruption, is a gift that few people have nowadays.

9 Bereavement can even affect the memory, and people will say they experienced a 'complete blank' for a period following the death. Almost every facet of life can be and is affected – only the scale and duration varies between people.

10 Thankfully, there are professional agencies that specialise in bereavement counselling and can be contacted through your GP. Nobody pretends that strangers are as good as friends or relatives, but they can often help people who have difficulty coming to terms with their loss.

Points to remember

a) People have different ways of expressing grief; there is no 'normal way'.

b) Talk about it, even if it hurts.

c) Don't be afraid to seek support from friends, relatives or your doctor.

d) Aggression is natural, even towards close relatives and well-meaning neighbours.

e) Allow yourself time to grieve, and avoid drugs.

f) Support for those left behind, and love for those about to die, can help make life better for us all.

---

5 Schizophrenia

Introduction

Schizophrenia is the most common major psychiatric disorder and affects about one per cent of the population of the Western World. It usually shows itself before the age of 25 and tends to last for life although there are excellent treatments.

The features common to nearly all cases of schizophrenia are:

a) delusions (abnormal beliefs not based in reality)

b) hallucinations (the sensation of an experience that isn't actually happening)

c) disordered thought based on the delusions and hallucinations

d) abnormal behaviour in response to the other three features

Schizophrenia often starts suddenly and may go on to produce a chronic (ongoing) illness. Nearly 80% of those who have a first episode will recover, but 70% will have a second episode within five to seven years.

Despite public fears it has nothing to do with having a 'split mind' and a very small proportion of affected people are violent. The majority are quiet people.

Symptoms

1 There are two types of symptoms which are divided into 'positive' and 'negative'. The main positive symptoms are:

a) restless, noisy and irrational behaviour.

b) sudden mood changes.

c) inappropriateness of mood.

d) disordered thinking.

e) feelings of being controlled by outside forces – having one's thoughts and actions taken over.

f) delusions.

g) hallucinations.

h) lack of insight – no awareness of the abnormality of one's thoughts, experiences and behaviour.

j) suspiciousness, which, in some cases, can become paranoia.

2 The negative symptoms include tiredness, loss of concentration, and lack of energy and motivation, which may be made worse by the side-effects of some drugs used to treat the positive symptoms. Because of these symptoms, sufferers may be unable to cope with everyday tasks, such as work and household chores.

Causes

3 Schizophrenia can run in families. When both parents have schizophrenia the likelihood of their children developing the condition is about 50%. There have been many theories to try to explain schizophrenia, and most of them have been rejected. People predisposed to schizophrenia can have the illness triggered (but not caused) by stressful experiences.

Complications

4   The major complications are to the quality of life, up to and including suicide. Treatment is becoming increasingly effective with less side-effects from the medicines used, but suicide remains a greater risk for people with schizophrenia than in the population generally.

Treatment

5   Early recognition of the condition with prompt treatment is very valuable and even life saving. There are now drugs which successfully keep the condition under control. Of the many types of anti-psychotic therapies, a Government body on clinical excellence recently recommended newer 'atypical' medicines, as they have advantages of older treatments, particularly in their side effect profiles. Other forms of help include:

a) *gently encouraging people with severe negative symptoms, who have become de-motivated and reclusive, to structure their days with achievable aims.*

b) *individual counseling that provides the chance to talk about the problems their illness has caused, how they feel now, and how recurrences can be prevented.*

c) *involving those living with, or caring for, those with schizophrenia in some of these discussions; the input and support of carers is an important factor in maintaining the future mental health of a person who has suffered an episode of schizophrenia.*

6   The modern outlook is a million miles away from the pessimism which once pervaded the treatment for the condition.

Action

7   If you think you or a friend may be showing signs of schizophrenia, contact your GP or:

Rethink (previously the NSF),
Head Office,
30 Tabernacle Street,
London,
EC2A 4DD.
Tel: 020 7330 9100
www.rethink.org

6   Stroke

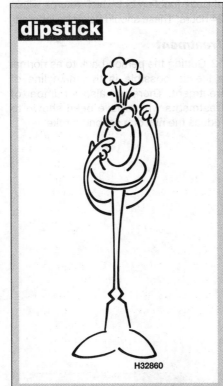

A stroke really is a major oil leak. Get any symptoms looked at right away

Introduction

Stroke is the result of damage to the brain, either from bleeding into it or from a lack of blood in one area of the brain, so that the function of that part is temporarily or permanently stopped. Strokes vary greatly in severity from a short period of muscle weakness to a more severe problem that can lead to death.

Strokes are the third most common cause of death in developed countries. They occur mainly in older people but one type, 'subarachnoid haemorrhage' affects younger people. About 1 person in 500 will suffer from a stroke each year in the UK.

There are two main types of stroke, cerebral haemorrhage (bleeding into or around the brain) and cerebral thrombosis (blockage of blood vessels in the brain, usually by blood clot). Cerebral

haemorrhage is usually the more serious and is a common cause of sudden unexpected death.

Symptoms

1   In cerebral thrombosis there are more symptoms than might be imagined because any function of the brain may be affected if the blood supply is impaired. The most obvious effects are:
a) *weakness of one half of the body.*
b) *loss of sensation on one side.*
c) *disturbances of speech and understanding.*
d) *visual disturbance.*

2   The first sign of a cerebral haemorrhage is usually a sudden severe headache. This is quickly followed by obvious functional loss such as paralysis down one side of the body, loss of vision to one side, fixed turning of the eyes to one side and perhaps a major epileptic-type seizure.

3   Smaller haemorrhages (and usually cerebral thromboses) produce less damage and there may be no loss of consciousness, but simply the signs of injury to the nervous system.

Causes

4   The main underlying cause of stroke is atherosclerosis. This is a disease of the inner linings of arteries in which cholesterol, fats and other substances are deposited in lumps called plaques. These narrow the vessels and reduce the amount of blood which can pass.

5   Such vessels are more likely to get blocked by blood by blood clotting (thrombosis) or by material carried in the bloodstream (embolism).

6   Cerebral haemorrhage, where there is bleeding into or around the brain, is the cause of the most serious kinds of stroke and is often fatal. Bleeding into the brain is usually the result of the rupture of a small artery, damaged and weakened by atherosclerosis, which gives way under the influence of raised blood pressure.

7   High blood pressure contributes to atherosclerosis and is the main risk factor for stroke. The bleeding can occur almost anywhere in the brain and the effect varies with the location. The pumping action of the burst vessel forces blood into the brain tissue which is disrupted and compressed.

5

Diagnosis

8 This is based on the symptoms and signs. The location of the brain damage can usually be determined from the effects. Specialised brain scans may be helpful in some cases.

Prevention

9 A good diet, weight control, regular exercise, regular checks of blood pressure, reduce the risk of stroke.

10 Smoking significantly increases the risk.

11 Advanced warning of impending strokes can sometimes be life saving. Often these come in the form of transient ischaemic attacks, sometimes called mini-strokes, where there is a sudden loss of body function but which returns within 24 hours. These should never be ignored.

Treatment

12 Getting the person back to as normal a life as possible is the main line of treatment. There are also a number of treatments which have been shown to reduce the risk of a second stroke.

Action

13 Make an appointment to see your GP.

Further information

14 If you would like to know more, look in the Contacts section at the back of this manual, or contact:

Stroke Association,
Stroke House,
Whitecross Street,
London, EC1Y 8JJ.
Tel: 0845 30 33 100

Chapter 6
Fuel & exhaust
(digestive and urogenital systems)

Contents

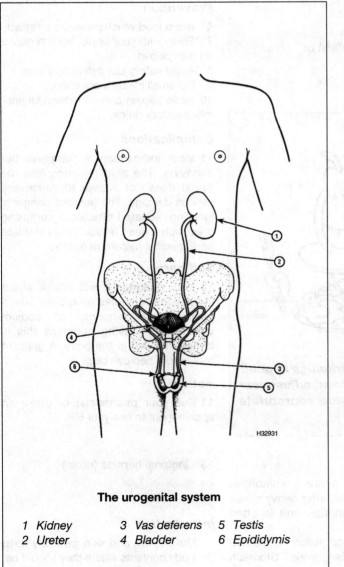

The urogenital system

1 Kidney	3 Vas deferens	5 Testis
2 Ureter	4 Bladder	6 Epididymis

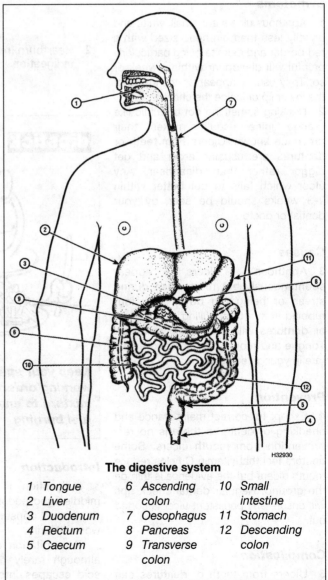

The digestive system

1 Tongue	6 Ascending colon	10 Small intestine
2 Liver	7 Oesophagus	11 Stomach
3 Duodenum	8 Pancreas	12 Descending colon
4 Rectum	9 Transverse colon	
5 Caecum		

6

1 Mouth ulcers

Introduction

Ulcers in the mouth are very common. The vast majority are harmless and will clear on their own. Unfortunately some ulcers may be more serious and need the attention of your doctor. There are different types of ulcer the most common of which is the 'aphthous ulcer' seen more in teenagers. Teeth with jagged edges or badly fitting dentures will also cause ulcers, particularly on the gums and cheeks.

Symptoms

1 Aphthous ulcers are small, white and usually less than pin head sized with a red border and despite being particularly painful will disappear within a week or so. They usually appear on the inside of the lower lip or inside the cheeks.
2 Drinking something hot or acidic like orange juice usually makes their presence known. Ulcers from teeth or dentures are usually larger and get bigger rather than disappear. Any ulcer which fails to get better within 2-3 weeks should be seen by your dentist or doctor.

Causes

3 Aphthous ulcers appear spontaneously but more often during stress or being run down. Constant rubbing from a tooth, filling, dental plate or dentures will also cause an ulcer. Tongue and mouth cancer is extremely rare in young people.

Prevention

4 Except for correct maintenance and checking of dentures there is no real prevention from mouth ulcers. Some doctors feel that vitamin C helps reduce mouth ulcers but the evidence is thin on the ground. Regular dental check ups will ensure any persistent ulcer is sorted out.

Complications

5 Ulcers from teeth or dentures can become infected making eating even more painful.

Self care

6 Aphthous ulcers may respond to salt water rinses. A mild cortisone cream will speed the recovery. Avoid antibacterial mouthwashes or lozenges which at best are useless and may even make matters worse. Make sure your dentures fit properly.
7 Avoid using gels which numb the pain as it will only disguise the extent of the problem. If the ulcer has not gone within 2 – 3 weeks, see your dentist or doctor.

Action

8 See your pharmacist or dentist.

2 Heartburn (reflux) or indigestion

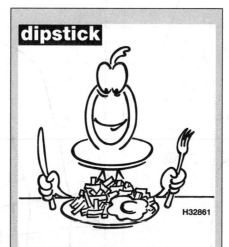

Keep your sparkplugs in good working order and adjust your mixture to ensure appropriate fuel burning

Introduction

Indigestion is more common in middle aged people, after heavy meals or alcohol consumption and is often worse at night.

Regurgitation or 'reflux' is painful although rarely dangerous. Stomach acid escapes into the gullet causing chest pain. It can be mistaken for a heart attack.

Symptoms

1 Symptoms can appear in the following ways :
a) *Vague pain below the ribcage extending into the throat.*
b) *Acid taste in the mouth.*
c) *Excessive wind.*

Causes

2 Classically after a heavy meal or drinking.
3 'Rich' food, often with a high fat content.
4 Excessive smoking.
5 A leaking valve at the neck of the stomach (Hiatus hernia).

Prevention

6 Avoid food which provokes an attack.
7 Sleep with your upper body propped up with pillows.
8 Avoid eating just before bed time.
9 Eat small meals more often.
10 Avoid aspirin and non-steroidal anti-inflammatory drugs.

Complications

11 Most indigestion is harmless but annoying. The acid refluxing into the throat does not appear to cause any serious damage. The greatest danger is ignoring repeated attacks or confusing them with a heart attack. When in doubt seek medical help immediately.

Self care

12 Your pharmacist will advise about indigestion remedies (antacids). Avoid taking large amounts of sodium bicarbonate (baking soda) as this is turned into salt in the body. A glass of milk before bed can help.

Action

13 See your pharmacist or make an appointment to see your GP.

3 Inguinal hernias (groin)

Introduction

Muscle, fat, and skin generally keep the body contents where they should be. Occasionally, either through a muscle

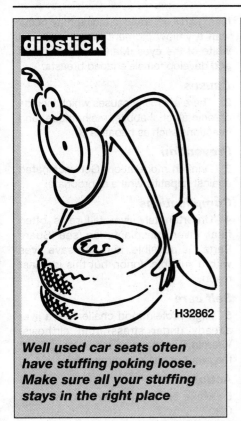

Well used car seats often have stuffing poking loose. Make sure all your stuffing stays in the right place

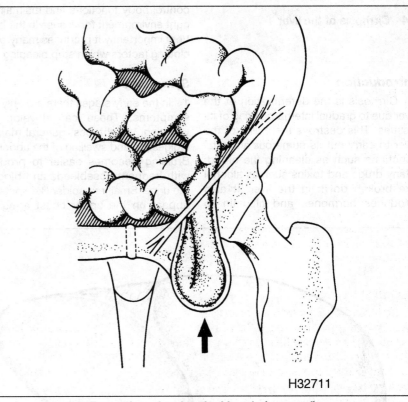

3.1 Formation of an inguinal hernia (arrowed)

weakness, strain or congenital problem some part of the body will squeeze through a gap and find itself where it really shouldn't be.

The most common form of hernia involves a loop of bowel which is pushed though a weakness or defect in the muscle of the abdominal wall. They are rarely dangerous unless the bowel becomes trapped, swells and cuts off its own blood supply.

An inguinal hernia is usually a loop of bowel forced through a weakness in the abdominal wall at the groin. For anatomical reasons men suffer from inguinal hernias far more often than do women.

Symptoms

1 Many men know when the rupture happened. Most describe a tearing sensation in the groin usually while lifting something heavy or even straining at the toilet. A small bulge appears at the crease between the thigh and abdomen. It can be felt better by standing up, placing two fingers along the crease of the groin and coughing. A light tap will be felt if there is a hernia.

2 This can get bigger as more bowel is

pushed thorough the gap, extending even into the scrotum.

Causes

3 While the male genitals are being formed a gap is formed in the abdominal wall to allow the testicles to travel from the abdomen into the scrotum. This leaves a potential weakness in the wall which may give way under strain.

4 Weak abdominal muscles and being generally unfit are said to increase your risk but not nearly as much as incorrectly lifting heavy weights.

Prevention

5 Hernias are very common (Gazza had two). Lifting is often a cause, so carrying heavy objects correctly is vital. If your work involves lifting heavy object or moving awkward things then ask for advice from your employers. Wearing a protective truss while lifting can also help, whilst keeping fit and maintaining muscle tone, especially the abdominal muscles, will help prevent a hernia.

Complications

6 If the loop of bowel is blocked it will cause an obstruction, and you will

experience pain. Your abdomen will swell and you may bring up foul smelling vomit.

7 This is an emergency not least because it can go on to become strangulated, cutting off its own blood supply. You will usually get some warning of this happening as the hernia becomes intensely itchy, painful, tender and hot.

Self care

8 Protective girdles and trusses can prevent the hernia from protruding through the abdominal wall. Thousands of trusses are sold or prescribed every year and they do work well for some people.

9 Even so, modern surgery is now so quick and safe that it is probably better to have the hernia repaired than risk obstruction or strangulation later on in life. It can now be performed under a local anaesthetic so almost all age groups can be successfully and safely treated.

Action

10 Make an appointment to see your GP.

6

4 Cirrhosis of the liver

Introduction

Cirrhosis is the deterioration of the liver due to gradual internal scarring of its tissues. This destroys the ability of the liver to carry out its numerous and vital functions such as cleaning the blood. Many drugs and toxins such as alcohol are broken down in the liver. It also produces hormones and albumin to control body functions and maintain the right environment for tissues in the body. Very importantly it produces many of the clotting factors which stop bleeding

Symptoms

1 In the early stages there are only mild symptoms. These can develop into vomiting, weight loss, general malaise, indigestion and swelling of the abdomen. Bruising becomes easier to produce, with frequent nosebleeds and blood in the urine. Small red spider like spots can appear on the upper chest arms and face. Later on, frank jaundice may occur with a yellow pigment in the skin and white of the eyes. Men lose their libido and develop female shaped breasts.

Causes

2 There are many causes which include chronic alcohol abuse, malnutrition, and infections such as hepatitis B.

Prevention

3 Drink in moderation. Get vaccinated against hepatitis where appropriate.

Complications

4 Unfortunately liver failure is often fatal. Liver transplantation (see 'Spare Parts') is possible, and can save lives with a suitable donor, but this is a last resort.

Self care

5 High-protein food challenges a liver already under stress from cirrhosis. Vitamin B complexes may help protect the liver but this is controversial.

Action

6 Make an appointment to see your GP.

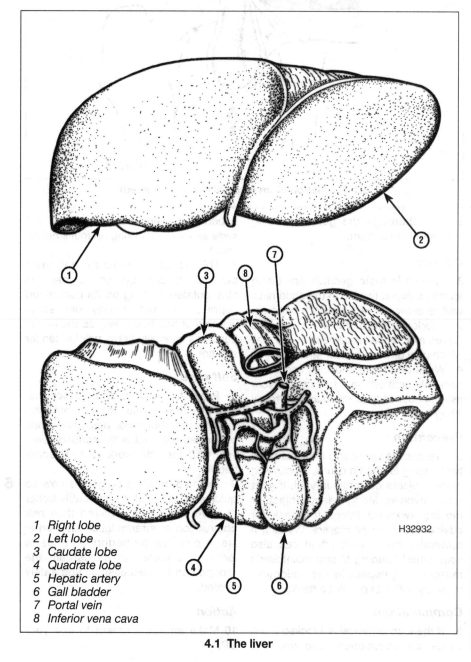

1 Right lobe
2 Left lobe
3 Caudate lobe
4 Quadrate lobe
5 Hepatic artery
6 Gall bladder
7 Portal vein
8 Inferior vena cava

H32932

4.1 The liver

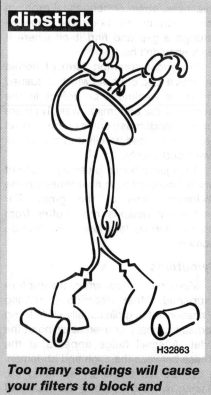

dipstick

H32863

Too many soakings will cause your filters to block and corrode. Try to drink in moderation

5 Diabetes

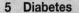
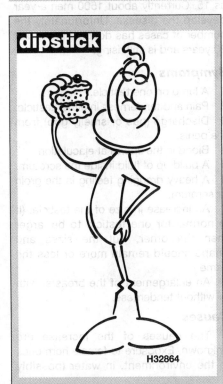

Diabetes is about processing sugar. You can't always have your cake and eat it

Introduction

Sugar in the blood varies between certain fairly narrow limits. Because people with diabetes have little or no insulin (a hormone that breaks down sugar), there is a constant tendency for the blood sugar levels to rise. An excessive rise is associated with the over-production of dangerous acidic substances called 'ketones'.

Type I or insulin dependent diabetes, in which the man produces no insulin, affects about 1% of the population.

Type II diabetes, often called maturity-onset diabetes, is regarded as a condition in which the body cells don't react to insulin, or in which the amount of insulin produced by the pancreas is not enough for the body to function normally.

Type II diabetes can often be treated simply by diet and, if necessary, weight loss. This reduces the sugar demands but, possibly more important, it also makes lowered demands on the insulin supply. Other cases require oral anti-diabetic drugs which stimulate the pancreas to produce more insulin.

Diabetes UK estimate there are 1 million people in the UK with diabetes, and another 1 million as yet undiagnosed.

Symptoms

1 Thirst, excessive urine and in type I diabetes, weight loss are the major symptoms.

Causes

2 Diabetes is caused by the failure of the specialised pancreas cells called islet cells to produce the hormone insulin. Insulin is essential for the building up of important large molecules, such as fats, proteins and glycogen, from small molecules such as glucose and amino acids and for the uptake of glucose for energy by cells such as muscle cells.

Diagnosis

4 Diabetes is diagnosed by finding sugar in the urine, and by testing the levels of blood sugar at different times of day.

Prevention

5 At present it is not possible to prevent type I diabetes.
6 The risk of type II diabetes can be greatly reduced by eating less so as to avoid obesity. Put simply, fat is not just a feminist issue, it's a diabetes issue.

Complications

7 Hypoglycaemia is an abnormally low level of sugar (glucose) in the blood. This is a dangerous state as the brain is totally dependent on a constant supply of glucose as fuel. Hypoglycaemia occurs when there is a failure of balance between insulin dosage, food intake and energy expenditure
8 Hypoglycaemia can cause headache, mental confusion, slurred speech, abnormal behaviour, loss of memory, numbness, double vision, temporary paralysis, fits, coma and death. The pulse is rapid, there is trembling, faintness and palpitations, and there may be profuse sweating.
9 The diabetic's behaviour is often irrational and disorderly and may be mistaken for drunkenness. The most common cause of hypoglycaemia is a relative overdose of insulin. The dose taken may be the same as normal but the carbohydrate intake may have been reduced or the amount of exertion increased so that fuel is used up faster than normal.
10 The immediate treatment is to take sugar and this will usually end an episode. Those with insulin dependent diabetes should always carry readily digested sugar or some other complex carbohydrate such as a biscuit, which takes longer to digest to prevent a sudden relapse. The drop in blood sugar can also be caused by over-dosage with oral hypoglycaemic drugs.
11 Glucagon is a protein hormone produced by the islet cells of the pancreas, which has an effect opposite to that of insulin. By causing glycogen, stored in the liver, to break down to glucose, it increases the amount of sugar in the bloodstream.
12 Poorly controlled diabetes can lead to eye, kidney and heart problems as well as erectile dysfunction. For example, diabetic retinopathy (a disorder, caused by diabetes, that affects the eyes) is the most common cause of blindness in the UK adult population.

Treatment

13 Any form of diabetes can be effectively managed so it doesn't seriously affect your life. Look at Sir Steve Redgrave, having diabetes hasn't stopped him achieving his goals.
14 Type I diabetes is treated with insulin injections and diet and exercise control, all monitored by frequent checks of the blood sugar levels. Pancreatic or islet cell transplantation is still experimental but there have been major advances.
15 Type II diabetes is treated by weight loss, diet control, oral hypoglycaemic drugs and also insulin injections.

Action

16 Make an appointment to see your GP.

Further Information

17 If you would like to know more, look in the Contacts section at the back of this manual, or contact:
Diabetes UK,
10 Parkway,
London,
NW1 7AA.
Tel: 020 7424 1030

6

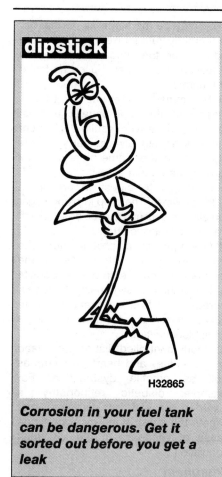

dipstick

H32865

Corrosion in your fuel tank can be dangerous. Get it sorted out before you get a leak

6 Peptic ulcers

Introduction

There are two main types of peptic ulcers, gastric and duodenal. Both affect the lining of the stomach and are more common in people over 40 years. Prolonged use of high doses of steroids, e.g. for asthma or rheumatic conditions, can cause a gastric ulcer. Even relatively small doses of anti-inflammatory drugs can lead to an ulcer in the stomach in people who are susceptible. Duodenal ulcers are more common in men. They heal more easily than the gastric variety and usually develop just at the beginning of the duodenum.

Symptoms

1 The symptoms of peptic ulcers tend to overlap, but a fairly general pattern is recognised:

Gastric ulcers

2 Constant pain or cramps can occur which are particularly bad after eating (eating tends to settle pain in a duodenal ulcer). Indigestion remedies (antacids) often settle the pain but it invariably returns. Belching is common and embarrassing. Vomiting can occur.

Duodenal ulcers

3 Most people know they have developed a duodenal ulcer at around 2 am when they wake with a pain like a red hot poker just above the belly button. Drinking milk can help, but hot spicy foods make it much worse. Eating small amounts of food often relieves the pain.

Causes

4 Ulcers may be caused by a bacterium called Helicobacter that lives in the stomach. Your doctor can check for this. Stress, smoking and alcohol abuse may also be causes.

Prevention

5 Avoid smoking and excessive alcohol. Milk and indigestion remedies (antacids) do help but only give temporary relief.

Complications

6 Call your doctor if there is:
  a) *red blood or brown soil-like blood in your vomit.*
  b) *black tar-like blood or fresh red blood in your bowel motions.*
  c) *severe pain just below the rib cage.*
  d) *dizziness when standing up.*
  e) *a strong thirst.*

Self care

7 Most peptic ulcers will respond well to treatment with modern drugs which reduce the amount of stomach acid. You can also help ease the pain by using indigestion remedies or antacids.

Note

8 If the pain has just started but is lasting more than a week, despite medicines from your pharmacist, call your GP.

7 Testicular cancer

Introduction

Thankfully testicular problems are relatively rare. Testicular cancer is the most serious. It represents only 1% of all cancers in men, but it is the single biggest cause of cancer related death in men aged between 18 and 35 years although it can develop in boys as young as 15. Currently about 1500 men a year develop the disease. Unfortunately the number of cases has doubled in the last 20 years and is still rising.

Symptoms

1 A lump on one testicle.
2 Pain and tenderness in either testicle.
3 Discharge (pus or smelly goo) from the penis.
4 Blood in the sperm at ejaculation.
5 A build up of fluid inside the scrotum.
6 A heavy dragging feeling in the groin or scrotum.
7 An increase in size of the testicle. (It is normal for one testicle to be larger then the other, but the sizes and shape should remain more or less the same.)
8 An enlargement of the breasts, with or without tenderness.

Causes

9 The causes of the increase are unknown. Exposure to female hormones in the environment, in water (possibly

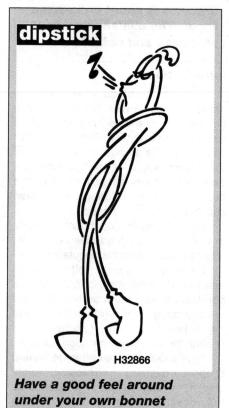

dipstick

H32866

Have a good feel around under your own bonnet

from the oral contraceptive pill in water supplies), or in baby milk have been suggested. In Spain and most Asian countries there has been no significant increase but we do not know why. At the same time sperm counts are falling across Europe and this may be part of the picture. Undescended testicles are a major factor (where the testicle stays inside the body after birth and will not sit in the scrotum). Men with one or two undescended testes have a greatly increased risk – one in 44. The condition can be corrected surgically, but must be done before the age of 10.

10 Your risk increases if your father or brother suffered from testicular cancer.

Prevention

11 For once men are positively encouraged to feel themselves, but this time to do more than 'check they're still there'. Self examination is the name of the game. Check your tackle monthly like this:

12 Do it lying in a warm bath or while having a long shower, as this makes the skin of the scrotum softer and easier therefore, to feel the testicles inside.

13 Cradle the scrotum in the palm of your hand. Feel the difference between the testicles. You will almost definitely feel that one is larger and lying lower. This is completely normal.

14 Examine each one in turn, and then compare them with each other. Use both hands and gently roll each testicle between thumb and forefinger. Check for any lumps or swellings as they should both be smooth. Remember that the duct carrying sperm to the penis, the epididymis, normally feels bumpy. It lies along the top and back of the testis.

Complications

15 Many types of testicular cancer can be cured in around 96% of cases if caught at an early stage. Even when these tumours spread, they can still be cured in 80% of cases, and large volume tumours can be cured in 60% of cases. Even so, late diagnosis increases the risk of a poorer response to treatment.

16 One testicle may need to be removed, but a prosthesis (false one) disguises the fact almost completely.

17 Treatment with radiotherapy or radiography may affect your ability to father children, but in many cases fertility is not affected. It is also possible to store sperm before treatment.

Self care

18 Too frequent self examination can actually make it more difficult to notice any difference and may cause unnecessary worry.

Further Information

17 If you would like to know more, look in the Contacts section at the back of this manual, or contact:

Orchid Trust,
Colin Osborne, Chairman,
The Orchid Cancer Appeal,
9 Grace Close,
Hainault, Essex, IG6 3DW.

TSE Testicular Self Examination Leaflets from:
McCormack Ltd,
Church House, Church Square,
Leighton Buzzard,
Beds, LU7 7AE.

8 Constipation

Introduction

One of the great British obsessions is with passing a motion every day. If this doesn't happen we think we are constipated. In fact there is no 'normal' number of times you need to go to the toilet. What we do know is that putting it off for too long can cause constipation. Thankfully, the serious causes of constipation are relatively rare especially in people under 45 years old.

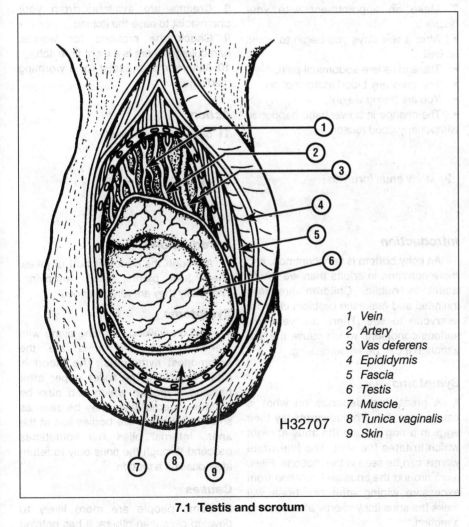

1	Vein
2	Artery
3	Vas deferens
4	Epididymis
5	Fascia
6	Testis
7	Muscle
8	Tunica vaginalis
9	Skin

H32707

7.1 Testis and scrotum

6

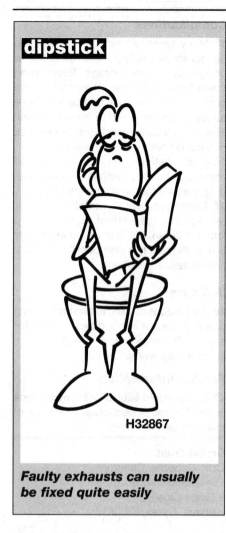

dipstick

H32867

Faulty exhausts can usually be fixed quite easily

Symptoms

1   A significant change in normal bowel movements with very irregular and difficult to pass motions. There may be abdominal pain and bloating.

Causes

2   Perhaps the single greatest cause in older people is a lack of activity. This is particularly true if there is some disability. Not drinking enough non alcoholic fluids and a lack of fibre in the diet are also major factors.

3   Many people do not realise that over use of laxatives can cause a severe constipation, particularly once they are stopped. Some medicines, particularly pain killers containing codeine, are powerful constipating agents. Stress can cause constipation, not least because it can lead to poor diet, but also stress directly affects the bowel.

Prevention

4   Most of the preventative measures are just sensible attention to the things that cause constipation such as:
  a) *Increase your fluids, particularly pure fruit juices.*
  b) *Increase your activity.*
  c) *Wean yourself off laxatives.*
  d) *Eat more fibre and fruit.*
  e) *Ask your doctor about the medicines you are on at present.*

Complications

5   Although it feels terrible, constipation rarely causes any serious harm. The big danger is ignoring the warning signs of something more serious and not having it checked out soon enough.

Action

6   See your pharmacist.
7   Make an appointment with your doctor if:
  • After a few days you begin to vomit as well.
  • There is severe abdominal pain.
  • You pass any blood in the motion.
  • You are losing weight.
  • The change in bowel habit happened without any good reason.

9   Itchy anus (pruritus)

Introduction

An itchy bottom is very common, and more common in adults than we like to admit in public. Children are less inhibited and make the problem clear for everyone to see. There are very few serious conditions which cause the itch although it can be embarrassing.

Symptoms

1   A great deal depends on what is causing the itch. Threadworms lay their eggs in a ring around the anus at night which irritates the skin. The fine white worms can be seen in the motions. Piles, tears around the anus and irritation from excessive wiping after diarrhoea will make the anus itchy shortly after passing a motion.

Causes

2   Other than those mentioned there is not always an obvious reason for itching although it is usually worse in warm weather.

Prevention

3   Wear loose cotton underwear.
4   Eat a high fibre diet to prevent constipation causing small tears around the anus or piles.
5   Use damp toilet paper first, then dry paper after passing a motion.
6   Avoid harsh toilet paper and strong soaps.

Complications

7   Constant itching can cause infection which only makes the itching worse.

Self care

8   Creams are available from your pharmacist to ease the itching.
9   Check the motions for worms, particularly if there is a night time itch
10 Ask your pharmacist for a worming medicine.

Action

11 See your pharmacist

10   Piles (haemorrhoids)

Introduction

Although the constant butt of jokes, piles are painful and annoying. Thankfully they are rarely serious.

Symptoms

1   Pain on walking or sitting along with bleeding from the anus are the commonest symptoms. The blood is often found on the toilet paper after passing a motion which can also be painful. External piles may be seen as small black grape like bodies just at the anus. Internal piles will sometimes descend through the anus only to return after passing a motion.

Causes

2   Some people are more likely to develop piles than others. It has nothing

to do with your preference of beer. Straining at the toilet, perhaps as a result of constipation, is well recognised. Standing for long periods may be a factor which is made worse by being overweight. Even lifting heavy weights has been suggested as a cause as it puts pressure on the veins in or near the anus. Contrary to what we were all told at school, sitting on hot radiator pipes does not appear to cause piles.

Prevention

3   High fibre diets not only bulk up the motions, they may also help prevent cancer of the bowel. Similarly, taking plenty of fluids, especially fruit juices, increases the speed of the bowel. Constipation is linked to inactivity so by increasing your activity you will reduce the likelihood of piles. Being overweight puts pressure on the veins near the anus in a similar way to pregnancy. Reduce weight.

Complications

4   Bleeding can occur which is more embarrassing than dangerous. Piles can

also thrombose (clot) causing even more pain and making it difficult to get them back inside the anus. Constipation can occur from not wanting to pass a motion because of the pain. This then makes passing a motion even worse. A vicious cycle.

Self care

5   Ice packs really do help.
6   Use a small car tyre filled with cold water to sit on.
7   Use a bulking laxative.

8   Use soft toilet paper.
9   Go to the toilet when you feel you need to, don't put it off.
10   If passing a motion is really painful, use a lubricating, analgesic cream obtainable from your pharmacist a hour before you go to the toilet.

Action

11   Make an appointment to see your GP. Although piles are far more common, some bowel cancers present late as they are ignored as piles.

dipstick

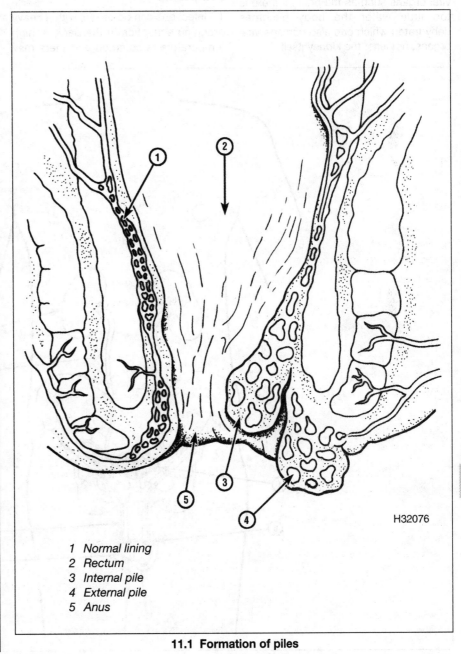

H32868

If you find yourself lost in Chalfont St Giles, go see your pharmacist for directions

1   Normal lining
2   Rectum
3   Internal pile
4   External pile
5   Anus

H32076

11.1 Formation of piles

6

11 Kidney infections & stones

Introduction

Kidneys are more than just filters, they also control blood pressure and stimulate the production of red blood cells. Their main role is to control the amount of fluid in the body and flush out toxins. If the body has too much water on board it becomes 'oedematous' and this can build up in the blood, damaging vital organs such as the brain. If there is too little water the body becomes dehydrated which can also damage vital organs, not least the kidney itself.

There are usually two kidneys, one on each side just beneath the back rib cage. They are connected to the bladder by long tubes (ureters). Sometimes there can be two ureters coming from the one kidney. In most cases this will not cause any problems but it can sometimes make infections more likely to occur. Kidney infections are relatively rare but can be serious. Kidney stones can form in the kidney and block the ureter which not only causes pain but may also make infection more likely.

Symptoms

1 Infections can be painful with a heavy dragging sensation in the back. A high temperature is common and there may be blood clots in the urine. Tenderness over the muscles of the back can also occur. Vomiting is common.

2 Stones can form from calcium or oxalate (a form of acid) and can be a sign of a mineral imbalance in the blood. Renal colic is described as the worst pain known to man and often requires very powerful pain killers to control. The pain typically radiates down from the back to the groin. Small pieces of stone along with blood clots may be found in the urine.

Causes

3 Infections can occur for no apparent reason but are also associated with congenital malformations of the kidney.

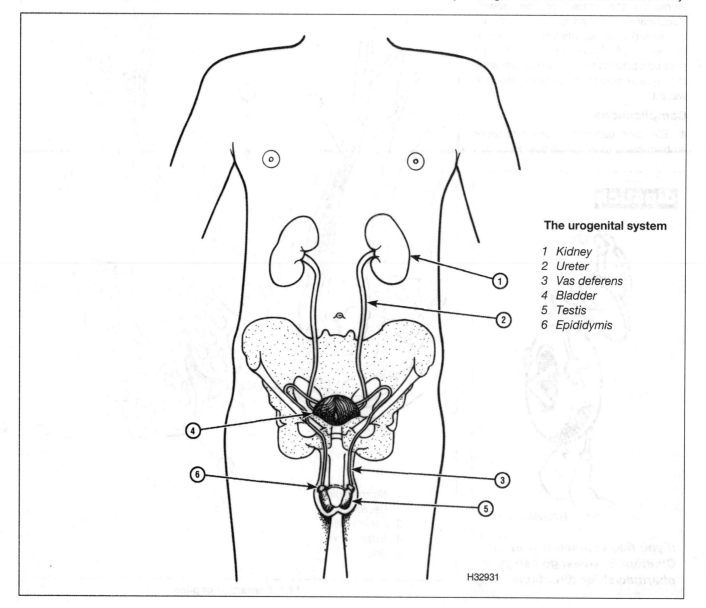

The urogenital system

1 *Kidney*
2 *Ureter*
3 *Vas deferens*
4 *Bladder*
5 *Testis*
6 *Epididymis*

H32931

Chronic dehydration is also a common factor. Reflux where the urine is forced back up the ureter is also a factor as is the presence of a stone.

Prevention

4 Both infections and stones can be prevented by drinking plenty of plain water each day.

Complications

5 Infections, dehydration and the back pressure from obstructions like stones can scar the kidney. If this happens repeatedly the kidney can cease to function and becomes a liability.

Treatment

6 Antibiotics will treat the infection, although it does tend to recur if the underlying cause is not addressed. Stones can be removed by various methods such as ultrasound which disintegrates the stone. In some cases a long wire with a basket is used to pull the stone down the ureter.

7 In very severe cases it may be necessary to perform surgery and if the kidney has ceased to function it will need to be removed. Fortunately the remaining kidney is more than capable of performing all the required tasks. If both kidneys have failed dialysis is required until a suitable donor kidney can be found. Thousands of lives are saved every year by people having the good sense to carry a donor card with them at all times.

Action

8 Make an appointment to see your GP.

12 Prostate problems

Introduction

Obstruction of the flow of urine by an enlarged prostate is common, particularly as we get older. Sitting at the neck of the bladder, straddling the tube which carries urine and semen, the prostate is roughly the size of a walnut and has an important job of providing nutrients and protection for the sperm about to make the long journey to the womb. Should the prostate enlarge too much it can obstruct and even completely halt the flow of urine from the bladder to the penis. When this is caused by simple enlargement with no involvement of cancer, it is referred to as Benign Prostatic Hypertrophy (BPH). Over 30% of men will have some problem with passing urine by the time they reach 50 years of age, yet only half of those men suffering will consult their doctor.

Symptoms

1 Poor urinary flow; frequent trips to the toilet even during the night. A persistent feeling of 'not quite emptying the bladder' often with dribbling after passing urine.

Causes

2 We don't know why it enlarges but there are certain triggers:
   a) *High levels of testosterone, the male sex hormone.*

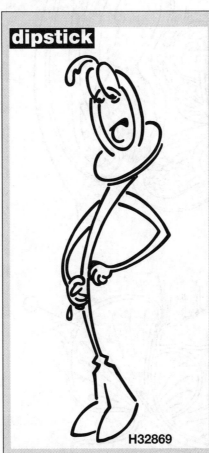

dipstick

H32869

Go and speak to your man mechanic if you're misfiring in the loo

   b) *An imbalance between oestrogen and testosterone.*
   c) *Possibly, low protein, high carbohydrate diets, high fat diets.*
   d) *Western diets.*

Prevention

3 Even though we are not sure of the exact cause of either benign prostatic enlargement or prostate cancer, sensible protection would involve:
   a) *Weight reduction if you are overweight. Oestrogen levels may be elevated in obese men.*
   b) *Limit animal fat intake, and reduce all fats anyway. It should represent about 25-30% of your energy needs.*
   c) *Eat at least half a kilo of fresh fruit per day.*
   d) *Increase your intake of antioxidants by eating carrots and citrus fruits.*

Complications

4 Urinary retention, being unable to pass water properly, can damage the kidneys.

Action

5 Make an appointment to see your GP immediately if there is any blood in the urine or sperm.

Further information

6 If you would like to know more, look in the Contacts section at the back of this manual, or contact:

Prostate Research Campaign UK,
PO Box 2371,
Swindon,
SN1 3LS
Tel 01793 431 901
www.prostate-research.org.uk

13 Prostate Cancer

6

Introduction

British men have a 1 in 12-lifetime risk of developing prostate cancer, roughly the same as a woman developing breast cancer. The risk is expected to rise to around 1 in 4 by 2020. There is an increasing risk with age. It is rare in men under 45 years. Currently over 10,000 men die annually in the UK as a direct result of prostate cancer.

Symptoms

1 Unfortunately there may be no symptoms until the disease is well advanced. It can also be confused with less dangerous conditions such as an inflammation of the prostate (prostatitis) and a gradual increase in size of the prostate without any cancer present (benign prostatic hypertrophy or BPH)

2 You may experience:
a) *Poor flow of urine.*
b) *Frequent trips to the toilet even during the night.*
c) *A persistent feeling of 'not quite emptying the bladder' often with dribbling after passing water (passing urine).*
d) *Blood in the urine or semen.*
e) *A severe backache for no obvious reason.*

Causes

3 We don't know the exact causes but there may be certain triggers:
a) *High levels of testosterone (the male sex hormone).*
b) *An imbalance between oestrogen and testosterone.*
c) *Western diets.*

4 Contrary to popular belief, prostate cancer is not restricted to the over 70's but is now becoming more common in the 50 plus age group. There is an increased risk of developing prostate cancer if you have a close family member who has suffered from the condition.

Prevention

5 There are no hard and fast rules for preventing prostate cancer, not least because we are not really sure what causes it. Common sense protection might include:
a) *Reduce the amount of red meat and avoid too much animal fat in your diet.*
b) *Avoid being overweight.*
c) *Eat plenty of fruit and vegetables as they contain antioxidants (chemicals which may prevent cancer).*

6 There is great debate over the value of screening for prostate cancer. The best test for prostate cancer is the PSA test which measures the levels of a prostate protein (Prostate Specific Antigen) in the blood. This is only of any real value in men who are experiencing symptoms. But when combined with a Digital Rectal Examination (DRE) (a doctor checking the back passage with a gloved finger), the accuracy of the detection rate of these tests ranges from 80%-90%.

7 PSA testing is most valuable when used on an annual basis since a series of tests can reveal those whose PSA is rising rapidly and are thus most likely to have prostate cancer. A new test, the PSA II test, will almost certainly re-ignite the screening debate as it measures the ratio of PSA floating freely in the blood and PSA bound to other proteins and this ratio differs amongst men with prostate cancer and those with BPH.

Treatment

8 Treatment choice generally remains between surgery and radiotherapy and there have been some major advances in both areas in the last 5 or 10 years. Hormone treatment may also slow down the growth of the cancer. Other treatments are being developed.

Complications

9 Surgical treatments for prostate cancer can cause erectile dysfunction (See Chapter 4) and incontinence.

10 The cancer itself can cause problems with passing water.

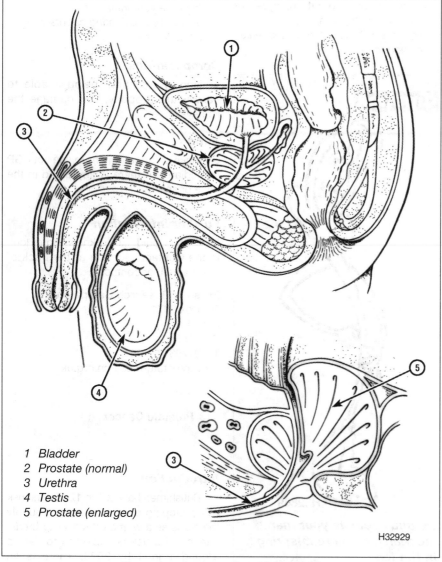

1 Bladder
2 Prostate (normal)
3 Urethra
4 Testis
5 Prostate (enlarged)

H32929

Normal and enlarged prostate gland

11 If the cancer spreads to the spine it can cause back pain which can be treated with painkillers and radiotherapy.

Self care

12 Keeping fit and mentally active is important. Prostate cancer tends to develop very slowly. Life can go on almost as normal. Although we are unsure if eating plenty of vegetables and avoiding animal fat will help to slow down the growth of the cancer, it will certainly help you in other ways.

Action

13 If you are concerned, make an appointment with your GP.

Further Information

14 If you would like to know more, look in the Contacts section at the back of this manual, or contact:

The Prostate Cancer Charity,
3 Angel Walk,
Hammersmith,
London W6 9HX.
Tel 0845 300 8383
www.prostate-cancer.org.uk

14 Worms

Introduction

Although we don't like to talk about it, worms are actually very common, particularly in children. It is not a sign of poor hygiene or bad living. Thread worms are the most common. They are itchy, embarrassing but harmless. Round worms are larger but less common. It is possible to be infected with worms from dogs and cats. Thankfully not so common, these infections can cause blindness. Tape worms are virtually extinct in the UK.

Symptoms

1 You may actually see them in your motions as tiny white/brown worms in the stool.
2 Itchy bottoms, particularly at night,

are the trade mark. The female lays her eggs just at the anus at this time, causing the person to scratch, pick up the eggs, and pass them on or re-infect themselves.

Causes

3 Infection with worms usually comes from contact with an infected person. They spread very quickly within a family and can remain in families for considerable periods of time without the family realising it.

Prevention

4 Wash your hands after going to the toilet or handling animals.
5 Wash your hands before eating.

Complications

6 Thread worms and round worms are not serious. Worms from dogs or cats can cause blindness, even in the unborn child if caught by a pregnant woman.

Self care

7 You can buy a preparation from your pharmacist across the counter but otherwise you will need a prescription from your doctor.

Action

8 See your pharmacist or practice nurse.
9 You should worm your pets regularly. Your pharmacist or vet will advise you.

15 Sexually Transmitted Infections

Introduction

Just one tip for preventing sexually transmitted infections, always practise safer sex. No ifs or buts. Use a condom whenever you have sex, because to be honest sexually transmitted infections (STIs) are a great leveller. They can affect you at any age, whether you're straight or gay, in a long-term relationship or with a casual partner. Symptoms don't always show up immediately, so you could have been infected recently or a long time ago. If you haven't practised

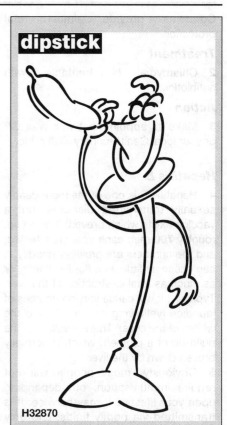

If you are going to have a bang, make sure you use your own airbag protection

safe sex or are at all worried, you can have a confidential check-up, and treatment if needed, at a genitourinary medicine (GUM) or STI clinic. Call NHS Direct on 0845 4647 for details of your nearest clinic.

Chlamydia

1 Non-specific urethritis (an inflammation or infection of the urethra) is a term which includes infection by chlamydia. Men suffering from this infection may complain of an intense burning sensation when passing water. There may also be a white discharge. It actually causes few problems for men, but can be disastrous if passed on to women. It is not only the single biggest cause of infection of the Fallopian tubes, leading to infertility and ectopic pregnancy (a potentially lethal condition where the baby attaches to the wall of the Fallopian tube instead of the womb), but can cause blindness and pneumonia in a child born to an infected woman.

6

Condoms provide almost total protection.

Treatment

2 Chlamydia is treatable with antibiotics.

Action

3 Make an appointment with your GP or your local Genito-urinary (GU) clinic.

Hepatitis B

4 Hepatitis B is one of the more deadly sexually transmitted diseases, but a vaccine exists which prevent it. Even so, roughly 700 men each year are infected, and the numbers are growing steadily. It can cause as little as a flu-like illness, or as much as total destruction of the liver. Typically, it will cause varying degrees of jaundice (yellowing of the skin and the whites of the eyes). This is caused by the build-up of a pigment which is normally broken down by the liver.

5 Obviously, most people will not require immunisation, but depending upon your lifestyle it may be wise. It is transmitted via bodily fluids, and only requires a tiny fraction of blood to transmit the disease. The virus can survive a week or more in the dried state and so can be picked up from, for instance, a razor. There is no way of knowing if the person with whom you are having sex harbours the infection. The incubation period, (how long it takes before the illness manifests itself) is six months from infection. Some people can even "carry" the virus and not exhibit the condition.

Genital Herpes

6 This is the third most common STI, and is currently uncurable. Herpes Simplex Virus (HSV) comes in two forms, HSV I and HSV II. Both infect parts of the body where two types of skin meet together, such as the corners of the mouth, and the outer parts of the genital areas. The virus causes crusted blisters, and then ulcers that weep a thin, watery substance. This substance is highly infectious, since it contains the Herpes virus. Coming in attacks which can last for months and then disappear for years, or even never return. You are definitely infectious during the presence of the sores, but it is possible to catch the virus

even when the sores are not present. Stress and other illness can bring on attacks.

Treatment

7 Anti-viral drugs can be applied directly to the affected skin or taken orally. They are most effective if used before the sores break out. This is signalled by a tingling, itchy, painful sensation in the affected area. Condoms with a spermicide appear to offer greater protection than those without. You need to arrange your sex life around the condition if you are having an attack as this means you are highly infectious. Otherwise, the use of condoms gives maximum protection for your partner.

Action

8 Make an appointment with your GP or your local Genito-urinary (GU) clinic.

Genital warts

9 Papilloma viruses, which cause warts, can affect any part of the skin. The virus can be transmitted by physical contact including sexual intercourse. Like the warts commonly seen on people's hands, they can vary in size from tiny skin tags to large masses. One in eight people attending GUM clinics has genital warts. Around 100,000 people are treated for genital warts each year in the UK

Treatment

10 There are drugs which can be applied directly to warts which will cause them to disappear. Genital warts usually cause little discomfort, although they are often itchy and may bleed with scratching. Use a condom to prevent catching or transmitting them in the first place.

Syphilis

11 Over the past 50 years syphilis has been rare in the UK, but now, along with most other sexually transmitted infections cases are rising. It is caused by a microscopic parasite, which is highly infectious. Most people are unaware of the infection, but if it is not treated it can develop over a number of years into a condition which can affect the brain. Women show few signs of the infection in the early stages except for small ulcers around the vagina so it can

go unnoticed by the woman or by their partner during intercourse. The parasite cannot pass through a condom, so this will give almost 100% protection.

Treatment

12 An injection of antibiotics will cure the condition if it is caught in the early stages.

Trichomoniasis

13 Causing a yellow/green discharge from the penis and vagina, this microscopic parasite lives in the urinary tract and usually causes pain when passing water.

Treatment

14 The parasite is sensitive to antibiotics.

Gonorrhoea

15 Caused by a bacterium, this disease often gives few symptoms, leading to common misdiagnosed. It is commonly known as the clap from the French word *clapoir* meaning sexual sore but is not rare. It can cause a yellow/white discharge from the penis, along with pain on passing water. Most of the symptoms of infection start within 5 days of infection and include a vague ache of the joints and muscles. Although these disappear after a further 10 or so days, the person remains infectious. It can cause reduced fertility if not treated.

Treatment

16 Antibiotics are usually effective. Condoms provide almost 100% protection from infection.

HIV & AIDS

17 Following infection with the human Immunodeficiency virus (HIV) there are less white blood cells called CD4, thus lowering the body's resistance to infection. Although the virus only appeared in the UK in 1982 there are over 4,000 new cases reported each year with perhaps 10 times this number unrecognised.

18 Early stages of infection generally go unnoticed and it needs an antibody test from a blood or saliva sample to confirm the presence of the virus. A vague non-specific illness similar to flu sometimes follows the infection at around 6 to 7 weeks later. A variable period of time, years even, can then pass completely symptom free. The occurrence of oral thrush, persistent herpes (cold sores) or strange chest infections which clear only slowly with treatment are ominous signs of the body's declining ability to fight off other infections.

19 Body fluids are often cited as the carrier of the virus. Actually this can be narrowed down to blood, semen and saliva. Although the risk of infection from saliva is extremely small it makes sense to avoid obvious risks such as oral sex without adequate protection. The main routes of infection are:

a) *Sexual transmission via blood from small cuts either in the mouth (oral sex), vagina, anus or penis. Sexual orientation is not exclusive, with both gay and straight men at risk.*

b) *Blood transfusion in countries with poor medical resources is still a risk. You can buy a travel kit from your GP.*

c) *Sharing dirty needles or even razor blades.*

20 According to the World Health Organisation (WHO) up to 90 per cent of those people infected in the World contracted HIV through heterosexual sex. Dental dams and male and female condoms, particularly those containing spermicide, give a high degree of protection both to you and to your partner.

21 Although extra lubrication is often required, do not use oil-based lubricants such as petroleum jelly or baby oil. They will damage the condom. There are water-based lubricants available. If you are not sure, ask the chemist, they will not be embarrassed to give advice.

Treatment

22 It is not all doom and gloom. New treatments are significantly extending life expectancy. Even so, the name of the game is prevention.

Action

23 You can attend either your own doctor or the local genitourinary medical clinic (GUM), which is located at one of the major hospitals in your area. Confidentiality is all-important at these clinics but you will need to be honest with the doctor. You can give a false name or remain anonymous if you feel more comfortable.

6

Chapter 7
Clutch, transmission & braking systems (muscles, tendons and ligaments)

Contents

1 Cramp

Introduction

Most of us will suffer cramp at some time. Muscle spasm which lasts for a few minutes most often occurs in the lower legs and feet. Lack of oxygen may be a factor but in most cases there appears to be no real reason although it happens more often while lying in bed.

Unfortunately there are some serious conditions which will cause repeated attacks of cramp particularly when walking.

Symptoms

1 There is a warning tightness of the muscle with a small degree of pain. Movement at this point seems to trigger a full blown attack and the muscles tighten into a hard ball involuntarily. Indeed trying to move it only makes the pain and tightening worse.

2 Eventually the pain and tightness subsides but here is a feeling that another movement would trigger a fresh attack.

Causes

3 Over exertion, sitting for prolonged periods, for example on a plane journey, over-heating, dehydration and exercising with a full stomach are all proposed causes of cramp.

4 In each of these cases the common factor is poor blood supply or over exertion. 'Normal' cramp can happen without any of these factors being present.

7

Prevention

5 Avoiding each of the causes shown above is the only real prevention. Warm up exercises before strenuous activity such as running or swimming will not only help avoid cramp, they will also prevent tendon injury.

Complications

6 Forcing a limb, foot or toe to move against the cramp can tear the muscle or its ligaments.

Self care

7 Cramp will eventually disappear on its own but can be helped by gentle massage of the affected muscle and gradual movement of the affected limb.

Action

8 If you are regularly suffering from cramp in any muscle you should make an appointment with your doctor.

2 Repetitive strain injuries RSI (tendonitis)

Introduction

First we had tennis elbow. Now with the explosion in the use of computers, repetitive strain injuries are more commonly associated with the wrists and fingers. In truth there were always a large number of people suffering from this often distressing and even debilitating condition. Musicians, particularly string instrumentalists, were well recognised to be at risk. Other occupations such as carpenters, electricians and nurses can suffer from tendon injury through repetitive movement.

Symptoms

1 It's not that difficult to tell if you have RSI. Generally the pain gets steadily worse as the day goes on. During your days off the pain eases only to come back again when you return to work. As the condition progresses you may find it difficult to move a finger, hand or arm.
2 In severe cases it may progress to tenosynovitis and you will feel a crackling sensation as you move a joint. It may even stick in one place only to suddenly move as you try harder to move it.

Causes

3 Tendons move inside a lubricated sheath not unlike an old brake cable. Either from injury or repetitive movement the tendon becomes inflamed and moves as if it were 'rusty' and in need of oil.
4 Worse still, this movement further inflames the sheath which tightens onto the tendon causing pain. In some severe cases small islands of bone form in the tendon itself which can completely obstruct any movement.

Prevention

5 Alternating repetitive movements with others helps reduce the risk. Use exercises which are the 'opposite' of the normal repetitive movement.
6 Every few minutes lift your hands from the keyboard and flex them downwards (they are normally held in a slightly backwards position, even at rest.
7 Use a keyboard which keeps your hands in the correct position. Similarly for people using instruments or tools such as screwdrivers. Either spend a few minutes during a job rotating your wrists and elbow in the opposite direction to the repetitive movement.
8 Consider an electric tool which eliminates the repetitive movement altogether.

Complications

9 Most people will find RSI simply a nuisance but for some it can mean the loss of employment and serious disability.

Self care

10 As well as the prevention exercises some people find great relief using anti-inflammatory drugs. Gels that you rub in may also provide some relief, but at least some of this comes from the massaging and warmth that it produces.
11 Applying warm compresses along with gentle massage can ease the pain.

Treatment

12 Steroid injection can give almost miraculous pain relief and restore normal function. Most doctors would be reluctant to repeat injections and it can be counter productive in that the person returns to the work which caused the problem in the first place. Eventually the pain returns and there may be more serious damage.

Action

13 See your pharmacist or ring your GP. If the condition is work-related, ask for a work station assessment; if this is unsatisfactory, inform your health and safety representative.

Chapter 8
Suspension & steering (joints)

Contents

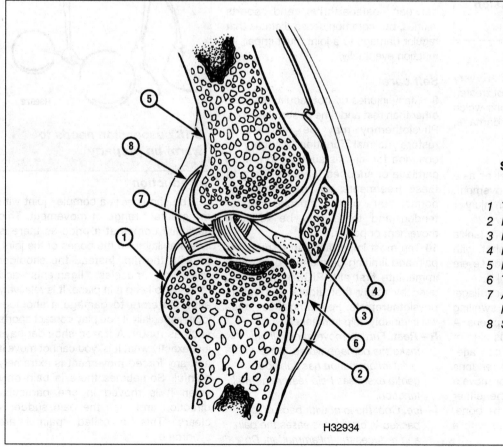

Sectional view of a knee joint

1 Tibia
2 Pretibial bursa
3 Patella
4 Prepatellar bursa
5 Femur
6 Transverse ligament
7 Anterior cruciate ligament
8 Synovial membrane

H32934

8

1 Sports injuries

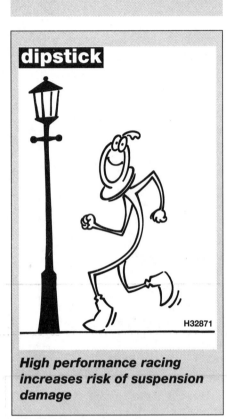

High performance racing increases risk of suspension damage

Introduction

Muscles, joints and bones are very susceptible to damage when not treated properly. They all have limitations which when exceeded will cause damage, sometimes permanently.

Symptoms

1 Some injuries show themselves as a gradual increase in pain on movement. This is typical of a repetitive strain injury or tendonitis (see Chapter 7).
2 A snapped Achilles tendon (ankle tendon) can sound like a gun shot, with immediate loss of power to the foot, severe pain and an inability to flex the ankle.
3 A ruptured meniscus (knee cartilage) invariably causes pain and swelling immediately or soon after it happens. A 'locked' knee is a very obvious sign of internal damage such as a torn cartilage.
4 Sprains involve damage to tendons and ligaments which stabilise or move a joint. These ligaments can be either stretched or partly torn from the bone. This causes pain and swelling with a restriction on movement.

5 In all these cases the joint or muscle becomes hot and tender.

Causes

6 Most sports injuries are caused by a force exceeding that which the joint, muscle or tendon is designed to withstand. It is often the result of a twisting movement under great force (torn knee cartilages) or excessive force to an unprepared or inflexible tendon (torn Achilles tendon). Simply twisting the ankle in a hole can tear ligaments and muscles which surround this highly complex joint.

Prevention

7 Warming up is vital. Many men snap their Achilles through sudden activity, especially if they are unused to exercise. Although some injuries are accidental and often unavoidable, the damage is reduced by having the joint kept flexible through regular exercise. It will also heal much quicker because of the improved blood supply.

Complications

8 There is controversy over the link between osteoarthritis and sports injuries, but common sense dictates that regular damage to a joint must impair its function eventually.

Self care

9 Many injuries do not require anything other than rest and time to sort them out. Physiotherapy may be required to restore normal function. Surgery is common for injuries such as torn knee cartilage or snapped tendons. Many of these treatments do not restore the normal state of the muscle, joint or tendon and there may be reduced movement or power.
10 The most important part of reducing pain and limiting permanent damage is immediate first aid. RICE is a system used by many first aiders and sports physiotherapists. Following these rules will invariably help immensely:
R – Rest. *Further movement will only make the damage worse. Once the initial inflammation has subsided gentle exercises help restore normal function.*
I – Ice. *Cool the joint with bags of ice packed in cloth. This eases the pain and reduces the inflammation. Do*

not apply ice, bags of frozen peas etc directly to the skin. Remove the pack after 5 minutes maximum. Reapply every hour in the first 48 hours.
C – Compression. *An elastic bandage will help reduce swelling. Make sure it is well above and below the affected joint. Take it off at night.*
E – Elevation. *Raise the limb and support it. This helps reduce swelling by draining the fluid away from the joint.*

2 Frozen shoulder

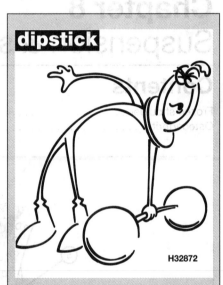

Stiff suspension needs to warm up properly

Introduction

The shoulder is a complex joint with the greatest range of movement. This flexibility comes at a price as there is little stability from the bones of the joint, as with the hip. Instead the shoulder relies on muscles, ligaments and tendons to keep it in place. It is relatively easy therefore to damage a shoulder joint, especially if you play contact sports such as rugby. A frozen shoulder says just exactly what it is; you cannot move it and any forced movement is extremely painful. Sometimes there is pain only when it is moved in one particular direction and then the pain suddenly clears. This is called 'painful arc syndrome'.

Symptoms

1 Most frozen shoulders result from an injury which didn't seem too bad at the time. With constant and particularly heavy use afterwards the joint becomes hot, painful and difficult to move. Eventually it is impossible to lift your arm without severe pain. It can also follow tendonitis as seen in repetitive strain injuries (RSI).

Causes

2 Most of the problem stems from the tendons which run inside a lubricated sheath not unlike a bicycle brake cable. Following a minor injury or with repetitive movement, the tendon and its sheath becomes inflamed. The point at which the tendon joins to the bone is also affected and may become very tender to touch. As the inflammation gets worse so the tendon is less able to run smoothly in the sheath and eventually it jams or is only possible to move with extreme pain. With painful arc syndrome, one part of the tendon is affected, usually on the muscle which is responsible for lifting the arm straight outwards away from your body. There is intense pain as the arm is lifted then suddenly it disappears once the affected part of the tendon clears the sheath only to return as the arm falls.

Prevention

3 All of the ways to reduce the risk from tendonitis apply for avoiding a frozen shoulder (see tendonitis in previous Chapter).

Complications

4 Untreated the shoulder may return to normal within a month or so, particularly if the work which produces the RSI is avoided. Unfortunately there can be a permanent effect on shoulder movement so it is best to do something about it when it happens.

Self care

5 Anti-inflammatory drugs from your pharmacist will help ease the pain. Massage and warmth also help. Physiotherapy is also useful and many physiotherapists specialise in these types of joint problems. Do not force the joint. This can damage the tendons, muscles and even tear the bone lining where the tendon joins. Avoiding the work which produced the RSI is vital, even if the pain has subsided with treatment.

Treatment

6 Steroid injections into the joint can make a miraculous difference. Unfortunately many people then promptly over use the shoulder 'to make up for lost ground', possibly causing permanent damage. Few doctors will inject a shoulder joint more than three times, many will not do so more than once and some refuse to do so at all as there is evidence that it can cause joint damage.

Action

7 Make an appointment to see your GP.

3 Osteoarthritis

Introduction

Osteoarthritis is a degenerative joint disorder. Although it is related to age, many younger people show early osteoarthritic changes, and the by the age of 65, about 80% of people have some evidence of the disorder. Osteoarthritis most commonly involves the spine, the knee joints and the hip joints.

Symptoms

1 Pain is at first intermittent and then becomes more frequent. Joint movement becomes increasingly limited, at first because of pain and muscle spasm, but later because the joint capsule becomes thickened and less flexible. Movement may cause creaking.
2 As the condition gradually gets worse stiffness increases and there is progressive reduction in the range through which the affected joints can be moved without pain.

Causes

3 The cause of osteoarthritis is unknown. Being overweight makes the symptoms of osteoarthritis significantly worse.
4 There may be a number of factors which include:

a) Injury.
b) Excessive pressure from obesity.
c) Over-use of certain joints.
d) Infection.
e) Damage to the joint nerve supply.
f) Other joint diseases such as gout or rheumatoid arthritis.

5 There is also some evidence of a genetic factor in osteoarthritis.

Diagnosis

6 The diagnosis depends on things such as:
a) The family history of any joint disorder.
b) When the symptoms started.
c) Where the pain is.
d) How severe it is.
e) When it is worse.
7 X-rays can be helpful.

Prevention

8 Eat healthy to avoid weight gain. Use gentle exercise to maintain muscle strength around the joint, to reduce problems.

Treatment

9 Weight reduction, if necessary, can greatly reduce the severity of symptoms. An exercise program designed to improve the general health and the health of affected joints is also helpful.
10 Immobilisation on the other hand, is dangerous and can speed the progress and worsen the outlook of the disease.
11 In osteoarthritis, drug treatment is of relatively minor importance because inflammation is not an important part of the process and infection is not involved. Non-steroidal anti-inflammatory drugs (NSAIDs) are often all that is required to relieve pain. Newer drugs are available which have less effect on the stomach lining.
12 Surgery to replace the joint is a last resource, usually considered before total loss of function occurs. A large amount of surgical experience of hip and knee replacement for osteoarthritis has now been obtained, and the results are usually remarkably good. Other osteoarthritis joints can also be replaced.

Action

13 Make an appointment to see your GP.

8

Chapter 9
Electrical system and sensors (eyes, ears and nose)

Contents

1 Nose bleeds

Nose bleeds are common. The vast majority are spontaneous, often following a cold or chest infection. Adults taking anti blood clotting drugs should tell their doctor or clinic as it can mean they may need to reduce the dose slightly.

Symptoms

1 Nose bleeds can look quite dramatic but they are rarely serious. They are generally painless and from only one nostril.

Causes

2 The blood vessels in the nose are very close to the surface. At one place inside the nose a number of blood vessels meet and bleeding from this area (called Little's area) is common.
3 In very rare cases it can be caused by a blood disorder.

Prevention

4 As there is generally no warning it is difficult to prevent a nose bleed.

Treatment

5 Cautery – burning of the blood vessels – by a surgeon does help but if you are prone to them it may well happen again.

Complications

6 Avoid swallowing the blood as it irritates the stomach, making you vomit.

Self care

7 Tip your head forward over a sink or basin, firmly pinch the soft part of the nose just in front of the bridge and allow the blood to run out of your mouth. It will stop bleeding in around 10 – 15 minutes. Once it has stopped avoid blowing your nose and cough gently for the next 8 – 10 hours to avoid starting a fresh bleed.

Action

8 If it fails to stop after 15 minutes, which is rare, you should ring your GP for advice.
9 If you are suffering from repeated nose bleeds make an appointment to see your GP.

9

2 Sinusitis (nasal)

Introduction

Although inflammation and infection of the hollow spaces of the face bones (the sinuses) is extremely painful, it is rarely serious. Some people suffer from repeated sinusitis while others avoid the problem altogether.

Symptoms

1 A great deal depends on which of the sinuses is affected. It can feel like severe tooth ache or a headache with tenderness under the eyebrows. Generally your nose feels blocked up and your voice has a nasal sound. It can last for weeks but most will clear up within 7 days.

Causes

2 Sinusitis is caused by sinuses which fail to drain though their ducts into the back of the nose. It often follows a cold or an allergic attack.

Complications

3 Serious complications such as infection spreading into the bone are now very rare because of antibiotics.

Self care

4 Sinusitis really does hurt, so pain relief is important. Use appropriate painkillers. Decongestants may help initially but over use simply makes matters worse, particularly when you stop taking them.

5 Stop smoking. (You may have heard that before in this manual but it is still good advice.)

6 Try inhaling steam from a bowl of hot water.

Treatment

7 You may be prescribed antibiotics by your doctor but they penetrate the sinuses very slowly and you need to take them in high dose for quite a while.

8 There are surgical treatments to flush out the sinuses.

9 See your pharmacist for pain relief.

Action

10 If the pain persists make an appointment to see your GP.

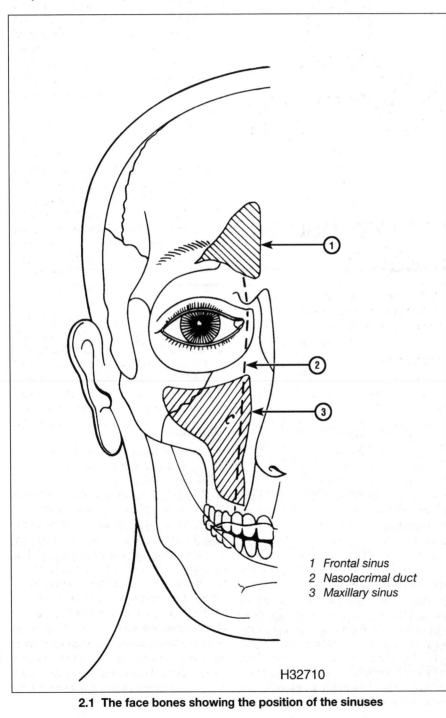

1 Frontal sinus
2 Nasolacrimal duct
3 Maxillary sinus

H32710

2.1 The face bones showing the position of the sinuses

3 Conjunctivitis (eyes)

Introduction

Inflammation of the transparent covering over the eye, the conjunctiva, is common. Infection, foreign bodies, constant rubbing or chemical irritation are all causes. People with allergies to plants or certain chemicals may inadvertently cause conjunctivitis by rubbing there eyes after handling the substances. In most cases the inflammation will subside on its own.

Symptoms

1 The blood vessels in the conjunctiva enlarge and the eye may appear 'blood shot'. Pus collects during the night under the eyelid and can matt the two eye lids

together. Bacterial infections, reactions to chemicals or allergies often affect both eyes whereas viral infections tend only to affect one eye, at least initially. Pus is much less of a feature with allergic or chemical reactions. Instead there can be a quite dramatic swelling of the conjunctiva producing a boggy plastic bag effect around the centre of the eye which remains unaffected. It will settle on its own although it can be treated with anti-inflammatory eye drops.

Causes

3 Bacterial from another infected person, often a member of the household or a school child can be passed on through sharing towels or even physical contact. This may also be true for viral infections although they also arise spontaneously. Grass and pollen will irritate the eye, especially if you suffer from hay fever. Wood resin, household chemicals, petrol, and many other common substance will also cause conjunctivitis.

Prevention

4 Using separate towels and face clothes while a relation is infected makes good sense. Wear goggles when handling chemicals. Take anti-histamines during high pollen counts if you are a hay fever sufferer.

Complications

5 Persistent bacterial infection can cause permanent damage to the front of the eye. Viral infections are more serious if they are on the transparent centre of the eye, not the conjunctiva.

Treatment

6 Bacterial infections need antibacterial drops from your doctor. It can take up to a week for the infection to clear but you can make things much better by gently cleaning the crusted pus away from the eyelids with a soft cloth and warm water. Antihistamine drops make a dramatic difference for allergic conjunctivitis and are available from your pharmacist without a prescription.

7 If there is any change in your vision, whether pus is present or not, you should ring your GP.

Action

8 If there is pus phone your GP, otherwise see your pharmacist.

4 Glaucoma (eyes)

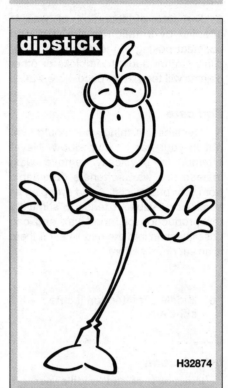

dipstick

H32874

Make sure your headlights go to full beam. Get them checked regularly

Introduction

The outer coat of the eyeball is tough but soft. It needs a steady pressure inside to maintain its shape.

Glaucoma is a group of eye diseases in which the pressure of the fluid (aqueous humour) within the eyeball is too high. This can happen in two ways. Either the tiny openings which allow fluid to leave the eye become partly blocked, or part of the eye moves forwards to block access to the openings.

About one person in 100 has glaucoma at the age of 40, but the incidence rises steeply with increasing age. By the age of 70, about one person in ten has significantly raised eye pressures. Chronic simple glaucoma runs in families and is more likely to occur in relatives of people with the disease. Only in the late stages will there be obvious symptoms. Central vision is usually the last to go and one eye may be completely blinded before it is appreciated that anything is amiss.

In other, less common, forms of glaucoma, the effects may be more obvious, with recognisable symptoms. In the most severe form the symptoms may be dramatic, with great pain and sudden loss of all vision.

Symptoms

1 Unfortunately, chronic simple glaucoma produces almost no symptoms until it is at an advanced stage at which much of the outer (peripheral) field of vision has been lost. Surprisingly, very few people notice the loss of peripheral vision despite bumping into furniture.

2 A less severe and less common form, called sub-acute glaucoma, causes symptoms that should be more easily recognised. These usually occur at night when the pupils are wide. There is a dull aching pain in the eye, some fogginess of vision, and, characteristically, concentric, rainbow-coloured rings are seen around lights. The condition can easily be prevented by the use of eye drops and is curable by a simple operation or outpatient laser procedure.

3 Acute glaucoma is hard to miss. The affected eye is acutely painful, intensely red and congested, very hard and tender to the touch. The pupil is enlarged and oval and the cornea steamy and partly opaque. The vision is grossly diminished. Urgent treatment is needed to reduce the pressure, so no time must be wasted.

Effects

4 If the internal pressure of the eye gets too high it will be higher than the pressure of the blood in the small arteries inside the eye and these will be flattened and closed. This can kill the nerve cells or fibres which detect light.

5 These fibres are concerned with vision at the extreme outer limits of our fields of vision and it is hard to notice that peripheral vision has been lost. This is because our brains concentrate on a narrow area around the point we are looking at. Many people can lose extensive peripheral vision without being aware of it.

9

Diagnosis

6 The best test is to measure the internal pressure by a technique known as tonometry, using a pressure-measuring device mounted on an eye microscope. This test is routinely performed by opticians when carrying out eye tests. Your eyesight is vital – an eye test costs a lot less than a car MOT.

Complications

7 A serious complication of undetected and untreated glaucoma is blindness.

Treatment

8 Glaucoma must first be detected, then treated. In most cases the pressures can be kept under control by regular daily use of special eye drops. If eye drops fail, some form of surgery will be necessary.

9 Laser trabeculoplasty uses a laser to burn several tiny holes in the outflow filter of the eye. This makes it easier for the aqueous humour to flow out and reduce the pressure.

10 Another option is trabeculectomy, an operation to provide an alternative route for fluid drainage out of the eye.

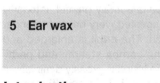

5 Ear wax

Introduction

Ear wax is very common and generally harmless, although It can affect hearing to some degree. Normal soft wax makes its way out of the ear and is removed by washing. Hard, or dried wax tends to accumulate.

Removal of wax by syringing can give great relief, but this should be done by an expert aware of the risks. It is better to avoid syringing, in case infected material should be carried into the middle ear through an unseen perforation in the ear drum.

Symptoms

1 Deafness is not caused by wax until the ear canal is completely obstructed, but this may occur suddenly if water gets into the ears lodging between the wax and the ear drum. Ear wax absorbs water and swells up.

Causes

2 The rate of secretion of wax is affected by irritation to the skin, and constant poking of the ears with paper clips. Cotton buds, toothpicks or other objects will tend to produce more wax.

Self care

3 The smallest thing you should ever put in your ear is your elbow. Never attempt to physically remove wax. Instead use wax softeners obtainable from your pharmacist. Avoid syringing as much as possible. It tends to stimulate the production of more wax and can pass infection into the middle ear if there is an ear drum perforation.

6 Middle ear infection (acute otitis media)

Introduction

Infections of the middle ear are common, particularly in children. Various theories attempt to explain this but we do know that the infections are not as serious as once thought. Even so, they are very painful and can cause a temporary loss of hearing. A recent cold or throat infection may have happened before the pain in the ear started.

Symptoms

1 Most people complain of a dullness in their hearing as if there was cotton wool blocking their ear. There is also a severe throbbing pain made worse sometimes by coughing. If there is pus behind the ear drum it may leak through a small hole not unlike a boil on the skin. Once the pus escapes the pain rapidly declines. It is difficult not to notice this happening as the pus usually flows out very quickly and has a strong smell. The ear drum repairs itself and there is very rarely any loss of hearing as a result.

Causes

2 Infections of the tube which connects the ear to the back of the throat the –

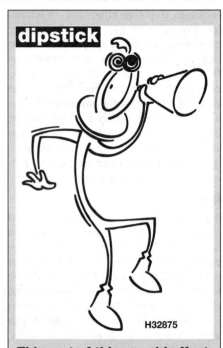

This sort of thing could affect your balance and roadholding

Eustachian tube – may help cause middle ear infections. This tends to happen during cold or flu epidemics. Its job is to keep the pressures equal on both sides of the ear drum, pressure builds up in the middle ear which is the main cause of pain.

Prevention

3 Some doctors feel that mentholated pastilles sucked during a cold may prevent the Eustachian tube from blocking but there is no hard evidence to support this.

Complications

4 It was once thought that middle ear infections caused permanent loss of hearing. This is no longer considered completely true. In the past serious infections of the skull bones next to the middle ear (mastoiditis) were dangerous and often lead to complete deafness in that ear. Thankfully it is now very rare although we do not know why.

Self care

5 Pain relief is the main treatment as antibiotics take a long time to take effect. Painkillers will reduce the pain and hard swallowing should be encouraged rather than blowing against a pinched nose to help unblock the Eustachian tube.

Action

6 See your pharmacist. If the pain does not subside or respond to painkillers, make an appointment to see your GP.

7 Loss of hearing

Introduction

There are many ways to lose your hearing. Terms like 'Boilermakers Ear' gave way to 'Disco Deafness' and will probably be known as 'Mobile Middle Ear' with the present explosion in mobile phones and personal stereos. Infection is another factor although infection of the middle ear and so called 'glue' ear are no longer thought to be a major cause of permanent hearing loss. Ear wax is a common cause of deafness, made worse by attempts to remove it with a cotton bud. This has about the same degree of success as trying to take a cannon ball out of a cannon with a ramrod.

Symptoms

1 Most people do not realise how much they depend upon their hearing until it is impaired or lost. Gradual hearing loss is usually missed or ignored until there is difficulty hearing speech. By this time the damage has invariably been done, particularly if it was caused by prolonged and repeated exposure to loud noise. There may also be a ringing or hissing noise (tinnitus) much worse when in a quiet room or at night. Less often there may also be dizziness (vertigo) although this tends to occur while the damage is taking place.

Causes

2 Prolonged exposure to loud noise is a common cause, particularly in industry and farming. Some viral infections may cause deafness and tinnitus. There are basically two types of deafness.
  a) *Conductive deafness involves the poor conduction of sound from the ear drum, along the middle ear bones (ossicles) and on to the sensory structure which converts the sound vibrations into nerve impulses for the brain to understand (cochlea). Diseases which attack the ear drum or middle ear bones reduce their ability to conduct sound.*
  b) *Perceptive deafness involves the cochlea or auditory nerve and this permanent damage is commonly caused by loud noise exposure.*

Prevention

3 Hearing loss is often joked about, and although some hearing loss is inevitable with old age, there is lots you can do, again in earlier life, to prevent going completely deaf. Wearing ear protectors and using sound baffles is relatively easy. More education is needed for young people about the dangers of using personal stereos, head sets and mobile phones with the volume too high.

Complications

4 Loss of hearing can cause accidents and potentially dangerous misunderstandings over instructions. It can be a terrible social barrier for some people. Some forms of deafness are accompanied by tinnitus which can be very distressing.

Action

5 Make an appointment to see your GP.

8 Tinnitus (ear)

Introduction

Tinnitus is a constant sound in the ears. About 25% of people with tinnitus experience musical noises, about 75% describe it as hissing, buzzing or ringing.

Nearly everyone has experienced short periods of ringing in the ears. This may be spontaneous or due to a loud noise, a cold or a blow on the head.

In established tinnitus, the sound is continuous, but sufferers are not always aware of it, so that it appears to be intermittent.

Most sufferers say that tinnitus is always worst in bed at night, probably because there is then less background noise. It is, to a variable extent, masked by external background noises that are usually present during the day.

Causes

1 Tinnitus is almost always associated with some degree of deafness and is related to damage to the hair cells of the cochlea of the inner ear. These delicate hair cells are the means by which acoustic vibrations are converted into nerve impulses for passage to the brain.
2 Tinnitus can be caused by any of the factors known to cause deafness, such as:
  a) *Nearby explosions.*
  b) *A blow on the ear.*
  c) *Prolonged loud noise.*
  d) *Fracture of the base of the skull.*
  e) *Tumour in the nerve from the ear to the brain (acoustic neuroma).*
  f) *Some antibiotics.*
  g) *Diuretic drugs.*
  h) *Quinine.*
  j) *Various ear disorders, such as Menière's disease, otosclerosis, labyrinthitis and presbyacusis.*
3 Explosions, and other nearby loud noises (acoustic trauma) are among the most important causes of tinnitus and deafness. After exposure to noise loud enough to cause temporary deafness, most of the hearing loss is restored, usually in a matter of hours; but some permanent loss occurs.
4 The causes of non-permanent tinnitus include:
  a) *Ear wax irritating the eardrum.*
  b) *Middle ear infection (otitis media).*
  c) *Glue ear (serous otitis media).*
  d) *Impacted wisdom teeth.*
5 None of these is likely to lead to permanent tinnitus.

Treatment

6 Certain drugs, such as local anaesthetics and others which interfere with nerve conduction, have been found to have an effect on tinnitus. Try not to concentrate on your own tinnitus. Distraction is the best strategy. Some people have found it helpful to listen to low-level music on personal head-phones. Others have invested in 'white noise' generators (tinnitus maskers). These produce a rival sound on which to concentrate.

9

Chapter 10
Chassis & bodywork (bones and skin)

Contents

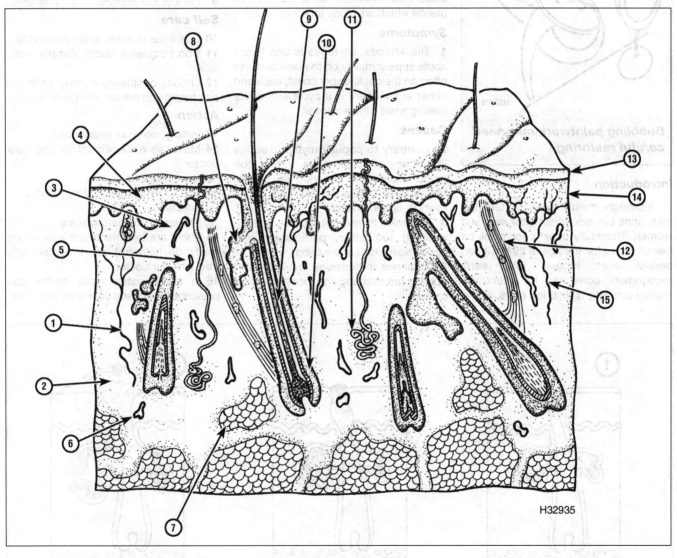

Skin components

1	Nerve	6	Blood vessel	11	Sweat gland
2	Subcutaneous tissue	7	Fat	12	Muscle
3	Papillary layer	8	Sebaceous (sweat) gland	13	Epidermis
4	Stratum corneum	9	Hair root	14	Dermis
5	Reticular layer	10	Hair bulb	15	Connective tissue

H32935

10

1 Acne

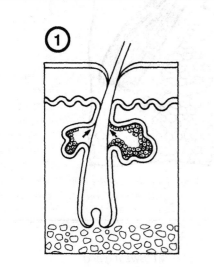

dipstick

H32876

Bubbling paintwork may need careful restoring

Introduction

Although mainly seen in teenage men, acne can also affect older men and women. Thankfully, most people will be free of acne after the age of 20 but it can persist even longer. With early recognition, acne can be effectively treated avoiding disfiguring scars. Some people are affected much worse than others but the way a spot develops is basically the same. Small glands in the skin (sebaceous glands) produce a oily/wax substance called sebum which helps protect skin and hair. The opening to these glands on the skin surface (pores) can block with a mixture of dead skin and sebum leading the way for infection. Pus builds up behind the blockage and the gland swells. Eventually the pressure forces the pus out of the pore.

Permanent scarring may happen with prolonged infection of a number of glands which are close together.

Symptoms

1 Blackheads, whiteheads and larger spots appear mainly on the face and less often on the neck, upper chest, back and upper arms. There is a cycle with spots healing while others appear.

Causes

2 Contrary to popular myths, diet has little if any effect on acne. Eating 'too much chocolate' is not a cause. Masturbation, blamed for just about every ill, is not a factor.
3 Dirty skin is also not a cause. In fact, washing too often, particularly with strong soaps can make things worse.
4 Changes in hormone levels around puberty are probably the most important cause.
5 We are increasingly aware of stress either causing or making acne worse. General ill health and being 'run down' undoubtedly affect the skin making acne worse and may even trigger it in the first place.

Prevention

6 Avoid harsh soap but keep your skin clean with fresh water.
7 Try not use products containing alcohol.

Complications

8 Scarring from infected spots.
9 Lack of self confidence in company.

Self care

10 Use a paper towel to dry if possible.
11 Don't squeeze spots. Simply wash well.
12 Lotions containing benzoyl peroxide can help if you are not allergic to it.

Action

13 Initially, see your pharmacist.
14 Make an appointment to see your doctor if:
 a) *It is spreading.*
 b) *The spots are getting larger and are infected.*
 c) *The spots are leaving scars.*
15 There are treatments available which really do help but are available only through your doctor.
16 In severe cases your doctor can prescribe a long term course of antibiotics.

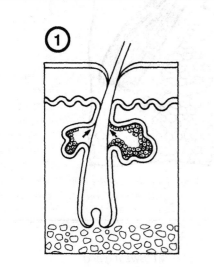
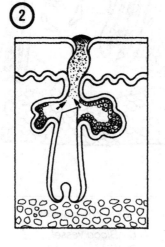
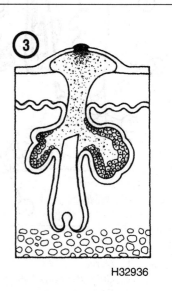

H32936

1.1 Acne vulgaris

1 *Normal hair follicle*   2 *Blackhead*   3 *Infected follicle*

2 Athletes foot

Introduction

Areas of broken skin especially between the toes are a sure sign of the fungus 'tinea'. It can actually develop in many other places on the body where it is called 'ringworm'. It prefers warm damp areas and is infectious but not as much as we once thought.

Symptoms

1 Red, itchy broken skin between the toes which can become white and boggy when damp.
2 A strong smell may be present, particularly after wearing shoes for a while.
3 Pain on bending toes, or tenderness over the toes.

Causes

4 Tinea is a fungus which can be picked up from swimming pools, baths or even wet floors. Sharing towels can transfer the fungus between people. Wearing trainers without socks makes it easier for infection to take hold.

Prevention

5 Keep your feet dry and well ventilated.
6 Wash your feet every morning and evening. Take care to dry them well, especially between the toes. Never use talcum powder.
7 Wool or cotton socks are better than man made fibres. Footwear with plenty of ventilation is essential.
8 Let your feet see daylight as often as possible.
9 Try not to wear trainers without socks.

Complications

10 Loss of skin can be extensive causing severe pain.
11 The infection can spread into the nails causing disfigurement and discolouration. The nails can become incredibly thick which can be painful as well as unsightly.

Self care

12 Simply keeping your feet dry for an extended period can help but you will usually need to use an anti fungal cream or powder.

13 Antifungal creams and powders can now be bought across the counter without prescription. Don't stop using until after a couple of weeks of fungus free feet.
14 Toe nail infections require prolonged courses (around 4-6 weeks) of antifungal drugs available only through prescription.

Action

15 See your pharmacist.

3 Boils & styes

Introduction

Boils generally form from infected hair follicles. If this is on the eye lid it is called a stye. When the body fights the most common cause of boils (the bacterium Staphylococcus) it builds a protective wall around the infection preventing it from spreading. Unfortunately this also impedes the body's natural defences from attacking the bacteria and a cyst, or boil develops. After a certain length of time the skin lying over the boil will breakdown releasing the pus. Carbuncles are just collections of boils very close together and are thankfully not seen very often.

Symptoms

1 It's hard to miss a boil. A painful red lump appears on the skin which

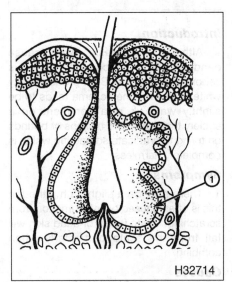

H32714

3.1 A boil generally forms from a pus-filled hair follicle (1)

gradually gets larger and more painful. The area around the boil is also very tender and slightly inflamed. After a few days a white/yellow 'head' forms which means the boil is about to burst through the skin to release the pus and ease the pain. Some boils will disappear without actually releasing the pus through the skin.

Causes

2 Being 'run down' or suffering from some illness which lowers your body's defence against infection can increase your risk from boils. 'Dirty' skin is not a cause of boils. Over washing with antiseptic soaps may even increase your risk.

Prevention

3 There is no real prevention against boils but if you are suffering from them often you should see your doctor.

Complications

4 Some boils can persist and come back again in the same place. This may leave a scar.

Note

5 Staphylococcus also causes a particularly nasty food poisoning which comes on quite soon after eating infected food. If you are handling food at home you should cover the boil, wash your hands and make sure there is no contact with your cooking. You are not allowed to work in any capacity with the preparation or serving of food for public consumption if there is a danger of contamination from a boil.

Self care

6 Once the head has formed you can encourage the boil to break by using warm water compresses. Soak some cotton wool in warm water mixed with a couple of spoonfuls of salt. Press it against the boil gently squeezing at the same time. Do not use the highly dangerous method of putting the mouth of a heated bottle to the boil then cooling the bottle to 'draw' the pus. It can cause infection in the bloodstream and may leave a scar.

More information

7 Persistent boils can occur if your body's defences against infection are affected by conditions such as diabetes or HIV. Long courses of steroids can also lower your resistance to infection. Some doctors will prescribe antibiotics but others feel that this may delay the natural eruption of the boil through the skin. Once the head is formed some doctors will lance the boil by cutting into the head and breaking down all the layers within the boil allowing it to drain freely.

Action

8 Ask your pharmacist for advice.

4 Corns and calluses

Introduction

People who always walk barefoot do not develop corns, simply thick skin on the soles of their feet. Localised skin thickening occurs over areas which are under constant pressure or rubbing. Classically they will form over the back of the toes or where the toes join the foot. Corns will also form over the ball of the foot. Calluses are also simply thick skin often seen on the hands of people performing heavy manual labour.

Symptoms

1 Thick skin itself is not painful. It is the pressure it exerts when pressed on by the shoe which causes bruising and pain. Calluses on the hands reduce sensitivity

Causes

2 The most common cause of corns is badly fitting shoes.

Prevention

3 Buy shoes that fit properly and try to walk around the house barefoot.

Complications

4 Constant bruising can cause a deep ulcer beneath the corn. People with diabetes should beware of this as they may not feel the pain and allow the ulcer to grow and become infected.

Self care

5 Wearing well fitting shoes will make the corn disappear. You can buy corn removal pastes from your pharmacist but the corn will reappear if you continue to wear badly fitting shoes. Pumice stones and sandpaper files can be used to reduce the size of the corn but over zealous attacks on the thick skin can

cause bleeding and infection. Soft rubber cushion pads can reduce the friction but may actually increase the pressure making things worse.

Action

6 See your pharmacist or chiropodist.

5 Dandruff

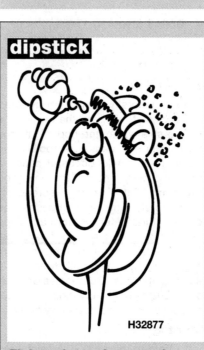

Flaky paintwork can make your car less attractive

Introduction

Although psoriasis will cause dandruff, the most common cause is seborrhoeic eczema. Both produce flaky white scales but the eczema tends to be slightly waxy. It is a comment on a society that we spend millions of pounds on trying to eradicate something which is completely harmless.

Symptoms

1 There may be a slight itch although this is often caused by inflammation from scratching. White flakes of dead skin will fall from the scalp particularly when combing.

Causes

2 Psoriasis is an auto immune condition (see psoriasis) while

seborrhoeic eczema may be a reaction to chemicals. There is an over production of skin which builds up around the bases of the hair follicles.

Prevention

3 Regular washing and brushing will keep the dandruff at bay but at the same time may stimulate its existence.

Complications

4 There are no known complications of dandruff. It is now thought unlikely that it causes any hair loss. Too frequent washing and brushing may be bigger factors.

Self care

5 Anti-dandruff shampoos do work although they need to be used over a long period. Once they are stopped the dandruff often returns. Avoid strong soaps and over use of hair gels.

Action

6 See your pharmacist.

6 Fractures

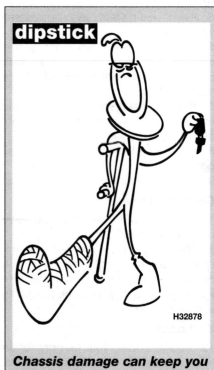

Chassis damage can keep you off the road for weeks

Introduction

Bones have many functions, not least producing new blood cells, but their obvious job is to support the body. They need to be almost rigid but not to be brittle. Bone is made mainly of a protein called collagen which is stiffened, strengthened and kept fairly rigid by the incorporation of mineral salts, especially calcium salts, and phosphates. Yet it is also a living 'organ' of the body often involved in complex metabolism and blood cell production. Without minerals bones would be quite rubbery, and far too flexible to do their job properly.

There is, of course, always a limit to the stress that a bone can take. And if that limit is exceeded a fracture occurs. Excessive force will fracture any bone, but a bone which has been generally weakened by a disease such as osteoporosis, or locally weakened by a tumour or cyst, will fracture under a smaller force. Such a fracture is called a pathological fracture.

Young bone, subjected to bending stress, often splinters on one side but merely bends on the other. This is called a greenstick fracture.

Symptoms

1 Signs of a fracture include pain and swelling, abnormal bending of the limb or part, skin discolouration and loss of movement. In the case of a fracture of a large bone, such as the thigh bone, the femur, the swelling may be very considerable, as a large volume of blood may be lost into the muscles and the spaces between them. This may be a cause of important complications.

Causes

2 The usual cause of a fracture is a heavy fall or other impact. People with osteoporosis (brittle bones) suffer fractures more easily (See Section 9 - Osteoporosis).

Diagnosis

3 Most fractures are easily diagnosed on the basis of the history and the symptoms, and are confirmed by X-ray.

Prevention

4 Sticks and stones do break our bones. Although fractures may be a part of the risk of living active and healthy lives, this risk can be minimised by taking precautions such as wearing the correct protective clothing. If you or anyone else is unlucky enough to suffer a bone fracture, make sure you've read the roadside repairs for broken bones in Chapter 1.

Complications

5 Osteomyelitis is an infection of bone and bone marrow that can also result from an open (compound) fracture. For this reason compound fractures require careful management in hospital by an expert. Intensive antibiotic treatment is necessary if the condition is not to become long-term (chronic).

Treatment

6 Fractures must be properly aligned. Once aligned, a fracture must be secured by some form of fixation until the repair is strong enough for weight-bearing. Various forms of fixation are used. These include:
  a) Plaster casts.
  b) Cast bracing with a joint to allow joint movement.
  c) External fixator.
  d) Sustained traction with weights and pulleys.
  e) Steel plates and screws.
  f) Long screws.
  g) Internal steel rods (intramedullary nail) for long bones.

7 Plaster casts are, effectively, bandages impregnated with plaster of Paris. Stronger versions now use resins.

8 An external fixator is a strong steel bar, placed parallel to the fractured bone. It is securely fixed to it by a number of steel pins passed in through the skin and screwed into the bone above and below the fracture site. The pins are attached to the bar by adjustable brackets.

A Transverse
B Comminuted
C Spiral
D Greenstick

H32937

6.1 Different types of fracture

10

9 Serious fractures often require internal surgical immobilisation by means of screws, nails or screwed-on steel plates.

10 Immobilisation may be necessary for a period of a few weeks to a few months, depending on the bone and the fixation involved.

7 Lice & crabs

Introduction

These tiny parasites live on any hairy bits of the body. Head lice live in scalp hair, body lice will live in the armpits while crab lice prefer the groin but will survive quite happily in your eyebrows. They survive by sucking blood from your skin which is why they are so itchy. Female lice lay eggs every day. The eggs hatch in eight to 10 days. Social status means nothing to lice. They are very common among children, and infestation has nothing to do with dirty living. They are completely harmless, but very irritating.

Symptoms

1 Itchiness is a common first symptom. The adults can be seen crawling about in the hair. Nits (eggs) can be seen attached to the hair shafts.

2 Inflamed areas around the hair shafts are common, usually caused by scratching.

Causes

3 There is only one source of lice and crabs: other people and their clothes. You can pick up similar parasites from pets but they don't survive long on people.

4 It is possible to catch them from second-hand clothes or wearing other people's clothes. Dry cleaning and washing generally gets rid of the adults and their eggs.

Prevention

5 Avoid sharing hats, scarves or combs.

6 Act promptly when warned of infection in the child's school.

7 Check all the family, lice like to move around and meet people.

8 Lice are easily caught from others, so avoid spreading lice by treating the whole family.

Complications

9 Although they are bad neighbours, lice and crabs do not cause any serious harm.

10 Scratching may cause secondary infection which may need antibiotic cream.

Self care

11 Keep the hair clean. Comb the hair while wet regularly with a fine-toothed comb. Use a conditioner. This helps to prevent the spread of lice.

12 The most effective treatment is daily combing with a nit comb followed by chemical lotions. Organophosphates are the mainstay of lice treatments, but there is some concern that they may be dangerous if used too often in young children. If in doubt, use only conditioner and nit comb.

13 As lice can stay alive for two days when they are not on a person, thoroughly clean clothes and hats which have been worn, as well as combs and brushes

Action

14 Ask your pharmacist for the most suitable lotion. There will be a local policy on the treatment of head lice.

8 Malignant melanoma (skin cancer)

Introduction

The 'wear and tear' surface layer of the skin is constantly cast off. Deeper in the skin is a layer of cells containing a brown colouring matter (pigment) called melanin that is responsible for colouring the skin. A melanoma is a tumour that starts in one of these cells.

About one cancer in 100 is a malignant melanoma. The incidence of this disease has doubled every ten years for the past 40 years. In children, melanoma may be present at birth (congenital) or may develop in infancy. In older children they are more likely to occur in skin that has been damaged by the sun. Certain other unusual

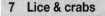

Rust spots on bodywork should be checked by an expert

conditions make melanoma more likely in children.

About half of malignant melanomas arise from pre-existing moles. Nearly everyone has pigmented moles, but only one in a million becomes malignant. Hairy moles hardly ever turn into malignant melanomas. Once you are suspicious of changes in a coloured skin mole, don't delay in reporting the condition for an expert opinion.

Symptoms

1 In white people, malignant melanomas occur most often on the upper part of the back. In people with dark skin melanomas are very rare, but when they do occur they are usually on the palms, soles and behind the finger and toe nails.

2 The signs of malignant change in a mole are very important to know. They are:

a) A change in shape, especially an increasingly irregular outline.

b) A change in size.

c) Increased projection beyond the surface.

d) A change in colour, especially sudden darkening and the development of colour irregularities appearing as different shades of brown, grey, pink, red or blue.
e) Itching or pain.
f) Softening or crumbling.
g) The development of new satellite moles around the original one.
h) The development of a light or dark halo or ring around the mole.

3 Report any of these changes to your doctor as a matter of urgency.

Causes

4 Melanomas are most common on areas exposed to the sun, but may occur anywhere on the skin. There is a definite link between sunbathing and the incidence of malignant melanomas. Probably the most dangerous type of sunbathing is a short, sharp period of intense exposure, either in a single day or over a short period such as a holiday.

5 Some white people are more likely to get melanomas than others. People with freckles and those with 20 or more birthmarks are at least 200 times more likely to get a melanoma than those with none of these features.

Diagnosis

6 Cutting out and examining the tumour is the only safe way of making sure.

Prevention

7 Avoid deliberate and unnecessary prolonged exposure to the sun. Always cover up. Particular risk factors for melanoma are fair skin and inappropriate exposure to the sun with burning. White skin in childhood may be especially susceptible. Every precaution must be taken to protect the skin against the dangers of ultraviolet radiation.

8 T-shirts or other protective clothing should be worn during swimming. Effective sunscreen creams (SPF 15 or higher) should be used, and it is best to stay indoors during the mid-day period when the ambient rays pass through the thinnest atmospheric distance and are thus most intense. Don't rely on sunscreen creams to protect you entirely. It is better to avoid

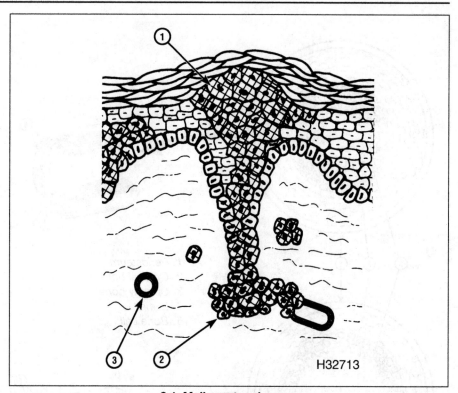

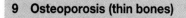

8.1 Malignant melanoma
1 Cancer cells in epidermis   2 Cancer cells spreading into dermis   3 Blood vessel

the direct rays of the sun by wearing a shirt.

Treatment

9 Melanomas are removed along with a wide area of normal-seeming tissue around them. Avoid delay in reporting any suspicious changes.

9 Osteoporosis (thin bones)

Introduction

Far from simply being scaffolding or girder on to which all the soft living parts of the body are attached, bone is constantly developing and changing its shape to meet the demands set on it. It produces blood cells and actively fights infection while at the same time providing support and protection for vital organs. For various reasons bone can lose its density and become light and easily broken. The constant replacement with new bone is affected by lack of exercise, some drugs and certain illness.

It usually affects people in their 60s and older and is unfortunately common in these age groups, with over half affected to some degree. Keeping bones healthy and strong while you are younger pays great dividends later in life.

Symptoms

1 Unfortunately there are no real warning signs that your bones are lighter and less dense. A chance X ray for some other problem will often be the first time a person is aware of the potential problem. Sudden severe back pain may follow a collapsed vertebra from osteoporosis. A simple fall can cause a broken hip.

Causes

2 There are a battery of causes of bone thinning. Immobilisation or lack of activity are major factors because the bone density depends on the forces it has to cope with on a regular basis. Long term steroids will also tend to cause bone thinning but the benefits of the treatment for, say, rheumatoid arthritis have to be balanced against the risk of osteoporosis. Osteoporosis is now well recognised in men and the gradual decline in testosterone, or at least in its

10

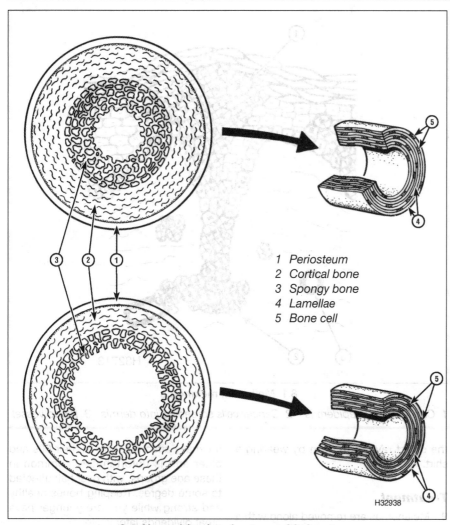

1 *Periosteum*
2 *Cortical bone*
3 *Spongy bone*
4 *Lamellae*
5 *Bone cell*

H32938

9.1 Normal (top) and osteoporitic bone

effect with age, may be a similar factor as with oestrogen decline in women.

Prevention

3   Some doctors believe we should be giving men testosterone replacement for the same reason HRT is used for women. There are now drugs intended to prevent osteoporosis on men. This is a developing area; ask your doctor for details if you are concerned.

Complications

4   The most serious complication is the increased risk of fractures. Hip fractures are particularly common although with modern surgery this will not mean permanent disablement.

Self care

5   Regular activity and a diet rich in calcium and vitamin D are the best forms of prevention. Eating bread, milk, oily fish, fruit and vegetables usually makes supplements unnecessary. Don't wait for osteoporosis to happen before changing your lifestyle as the damage will have been done.

Further information

6   If you would like to know more, look in the Contacts section at the back of this manual, or contact:

National Osteoporosis Society
Tel: 01761 471771
www.nos.org.uk

10 Psoriasis

Introduction

Contrary to popular myth, psoriasis is not an infection and you cannot catch it from anyone else or their clothes. The silver flaky patches of skin are simply cells which are growing too fast. Around 2.5% (1 in 40) of the population suffer from psoriasis which does tend to run in families.

Symptoms

1   Psoriasis is classically found on the elbows and knees and the scalp. It tends to spare the face. In more severe cases it can also affect the soles of the feet, palms of the hands, small of the back and armpits. The oval red patches are often covered with silver flaky scales which come away easily to expose the darker layers underneath. They are not usually itchy unless infected.

Causes

2   Psoriasis is an autoimmune condition where for some reason the body attacks itself. It is linked to other similar conditions such as rheumatoid arthritis. We now know there are various triggers which stimulate these areas of skin to start growing too fast. Stress, over work, changes in climate and even minor infections may be enough to start the process off.

Prevention

3   It is difficult to suggest any effective form of protection from psoriasis outbreaks. Dealing effectively with stress through both relaxation and activity instead of resorting to alcohol may be valuable.

Complications

4   The rash is not dangerous unless it is very extensive or is infected. When the rash appears on the hands or feet it usually forms fluid filled blisters which resemble pus. There is no infection. A small proportion of psoriasis sufferers, 6-7% (less than one in 10) will experience joint pain resembling that of rheumatoid arthritis.

Self care

5   Care and treatment depends on the severity of the condition. Sunlight appears to help some people which is not surprising as ultra violet (UV) treatments have long been used with moderate success. Other advice:
a) *Avoid strong soaps.*
b) *Avoid overheating by wearing light cotton clothes.*

c) If the patches itch, use a moisturising cream but do not scratch them.

d) Keep your skin moist with special creams called emollients.

6 Tar-containing products from the pharmacist can be effective, but do unfortunately stain clothes and need to be applied with care only to the affected skin.

Treatment

7 Your doctor may refer you to a specialist who can arrange treatment only available in hospital as an out patient.

Action

8 See your pharmacist or make an appointment to see your GP.

---

11 Ringworm (tinea)

Introduction

Ringworm (Tinea) can affect many parts of the body, particularly the groin and scalp. It is not a worm, simply a fungus.

Symptoms

1 It is most noticeable on bare skin when it is referred to as ringworm due to its characteristic appearance as a circular patch of red, itchy skin, which gradually increases in size.

2 There may also be red itchy areas around the base of hair shafts. With scratching, these areas can bleed and become crusted with blood.

Prevention

3 Keep the area well ventilated and dry.
4 Use a separate face cloth and towel – ringworm is infectious.

Complications

5 Bacterial infection from scratching is common.

Self care

6 Keep the area well ventilated and dry.
7 Use an antifungal cream or shampoo available from your pharmacist.

Action

8 See your pharmacist or make an appointment to see your GP.

---

12 Shingles

Introduction

One step up from cold sores, shingles is caused by a closely related virus. It is particularly nasty if the immune system is not working properly, during illness or while on treatment for cancer.

It is rare to develop shingles more than once.

Symptoms

1 A tingling itchy feeling precedes a painful rash. It is only found on one side of the body.

2 It can develop over the next few hours or days into a painful set of blisters. It usually follows a narrow strip of skin, common sites include the chest wall, face and upper legs.

3 A general flu-like illness often accompanies the rash and may persist after the rash has gone.

Causes

4 If you have never had chicken pox you are very unlikely to develop shingles which is caused by the same virus reactivated.

Prevention

5 Prevention is difficult, most people will develop the infection without realising where it came from.

Complications

6 Although sometimes very painful, shingles is rarely serious.

7 People who are suffering from any condition or medicine which lowers their resistance to infection can be quite ill.

8 If it spreads near the ears or eyes, or onto the tip of the nose, immediate attention from your doctor is recommended.

Self care

9 Simple pain killers can help.
10 Keep the rash area uncovered as much as possible.
11 Try not to scratch the rash. Ask your pharmacist about lotions to ease the itching.
12 Pain which follows the disappearance of the rash can be reduced by cooling the area with a bag of ice (don't apply directly to the skin).

Treatment

13 Once the tingling sensation begins it is wise to start antiviral medicine. It is important to start treatment as soon as possible. Once the rash is well developed anti-viral agents are of no great value.

Action

14 Make an appointment to see your doctor, especially if:
a) The outbreak of blisters occurs near your eye or at the tip of your nose.
b) You also have a sore red eye.
c) The sores have not healed after 10 days.
d) There is also a high temperature.
e) You suffer from some other serious illness.

---

13 Sun burn

Introduction

Although there is some controversy over the danger of exposure to too much sunlight, we do know that it can be harmful. Over the past few decades there has been a dramatic increase in the number of cases of malignant melanoma, a particularly nasty and potentially lethal skin cancer. Once considered rare, it is still increasing possibly due to the desire for sun drenched holidays. Australia has been in the forefront of educating people over the dangers of sun bathing.

Symptoms

1 Most people do not realise that they have badly burned themselves until later on in the day. The first sign of a burn is a reddening of the skin caused by blood vessels increasing in size to get rid of as much heat as possible. At this stage damage is already being done to the skin.

Causes

2 Ultra violet light (UV) can penetrate the outer layers of skin, especially in fair skinned people. It heats and damages the lower layers causing skin loss. The body responds by increasing the amount of melanin, a black pigment, in the skin which prevents the sun from reaching

the delicate lower skin layers. This is the 'sun tan' we crave so much.

Prevention

3 It's not too smart to go out in the sun wearing nothing but your union jack shorts. Never mind the crimes against fashion, it's potentially deadly. Use a strong sun block (SPF 15 and over). Cover your body, especially the head, with appropriate clothing. Never leave a baby exposed to the sun, even if the weather is hazy.

Complications

4 If the exposure to the sun continues the skin will form blisters just as with a scald. These blisters burst very quickly and the covering skin is then lost exposing red skin beneath. If this is extensive, a large amount of body fluids can be lost, a particular danger to babies and small children who do not have a large body mass.

5 Like any burn, skin damaged by over exposure to UV can scar.

6 Long term exposure to the sun causes the collagen network within the skin to become less flexible. This makes the skin lose its elasticity so it droops, folds and wrinkles very easily.

Self care

4 A badly burnt baby or small child needs to go to hospital. Treat sun burn like any other burn. There are lotions you can apply which will ease the pain but they cannot prevent the damage which is already done. Take plenty of non alcoholic fluids and stay out of the sun for a few days. Use only tepid baths.

More information

5 See melanoma (Section 8).

Note

6 There is no 'safe' exposure time. The rate at which you burn depends on the colour of your skin. Fair complexions are the easiest to damage with UV. Dark skin is the most resistant but will still be burned with prolonged exposure. Generally after 15 minutes on a first exposure white skin is already damaged.

Action

7 See your pharmacist.

14 Warts & verrucas

Introduction

Around 5% (1 in 20) school children will suffer from warts or verrucas. Warts and verrucas are less infectious than we once thought. Even so the link with cervical cancer needs to be taken seriously so warts on the penis should be treated as soon as possible.

Symptoms

1 Warts can appear anywhere on the body but are most common on the hands and feet. They can also appear at the anus and penis.

Causes

2 'Dirty' skin is not a cause. The Papilloma virus actually causes the skin to produce warts. There may be a

difference between the viruses which cause hand and feet warts to those which cause genital warts.

Prevention

3 Wearing protective footwear at public baths may decrease the risk of passing on or picking up the infection.

Complications

4 Most warts are not dangerous. Verrucas may cause pain when walking. Warts on the penis should be removed at a GUM (genito-urinary medical) clinic. They are linked to cervical cancer although their link with cancer of the penis is less clear.

Self care

5 Warts appear to have a limited lifespan and eventually disappear on their own. It can be a frustrating wait as new warts may appear as the older warts depart. Wart removal creams are available from your pharmacist. It takes great patience as repeated applications for more than a week are often required.

Note

6 Do not use wart removal pastes or creams on your face, anus or genitals.

Treatment

7 Some GP practices offer wart removal using liquid nitrogen or by burning (diathermy).

Action

8 Ask your pharmacist for advice. Ring the local genito-urinary (GUM) clinic if you suspect they are genital or anal warts.

Reference

Contents

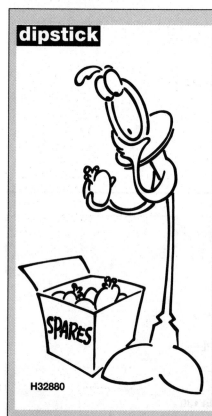

dipstick

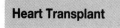

H32880

Parts are often in very short supply and don't fit all models. Always carry a Donor Card.

Heart Transplant

Introduction

Patients who need a transplant require a donor whose heart is still beating at death. Thousands of such transplants are carried out in the world each year. Most donors will be brain dead from a cause such as stroke or accident.

Why is it necessary?

Heart failure is progressive and often a transplant is the only option.

Poor heart activity can lead to brain and other organ damage so it is often the only option for survival.

When should it be done?

Most surgeons prefer to transplant before the patient is so ill they cannot be expected to survive the transplant procedure itself. This is a balance

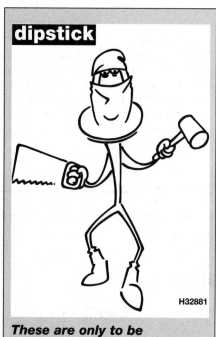

dipstick

H32881

These are only to be performed by expert qualified man mechanics

between the dangers of transplant against the inevitable consequences of the heart disease itself.

How is it performed?

Many transplants are in fact partial where the lower part of the heart (the ventricles) is transplanted. If the lungs are also part of the problem they are transplanted as part of the heart/lung transplant.

Results

The majority of people with a heart transplant are still alive 5 years later. A great deal depends on the original problem and the age of the person.

Future prospects

Artificial hearts and animal transplants are still experimental, but gaining ground rapidly.

Kidney transplant

Introduction

Many thousands of people have received a kidney through transplantation and the procedure is now routine.

Why is it necessary?

Most people can be kept in reasonably good health by using dialysis but transplantation can give a better quality of life. It is often the last resort after both kidneys fail to perform adequately and there is poor response to dialysis.

When should it be done?

Kidney transplant is now done much sooner if the quality of life will be better than remaining on dialysis. The critical factor is the availability of a suitable donor kidney.

How is it performed?

Most donor kidneys are taken from people who have died from accidents or from live relatives willing to donate their kidney to a relative. Human generosity never fails to impress just how much people value other people's lives.

Results

More than 80% of people receiving a transplant still have a functioning kidney two years later. There is a risk from infection and rejection but this is getting to be less serious than previously.

Liver transplant

Introduction

Many thousands of liver transplants have been done; a shortage of donors is the main problem. The risks involved in transplantation include:
a) *Failure of the donated liver to function*
b) *Acute rejection of the donated liver*
c) *Development of hepatitis in the new liver, mainly from one of a variety of infections*
d) *Obstruction to the release of bile from the transplanted liver.*

Why it is necessary?

Liver transplantation is the only chance for people whose livers are so diseased that they are no longer able to maintain normal living. In most cases, these are people with cirrhosis of the liver. Acute liver failure and primary liver cancer are less common reasons for transplantation.

When should it be done?

Transplantation is usually the last resort after all else has failed, so the person tends to be very ill but has no other option.

How is it performed?

In some cases a live donor may give a part of his or her liver for transplantation. The remaining tissue will regenerate new liver tissue. These cases are called 'split-liver' transplants.

A liver transplant is a complicated procedure involving at least a 8-hour operation. The diseased liver has to be removed. Connections have to be made to many of the large veins in the body, to the arteries supplying the liver with blood, and to the intestine for the bile duct.

Results

The results of liver transplantation have been improving steadily. Survival rate over one year is about 90% and over five years is 70 to 85%. Most of the deaths occur from organ rejection within the first three months after the operation. Patients who survive are able to lead a normal life and, in almost all, the quality of life is greatly improved.

Blood pressure measurement

Description

Myths surround every aspect of blood pressure. It helps to know what is being measured in the first place. Blood pressure (BP) is always written as two numbers thus: 120/80. Neither of these numbers has anything to do with your age, height or weight. They are simple measurements of the heart's ability to overcome pressure from an inflated cuff placed around the arm or leg.

How is it done?

As the cuff is slowly deflated, the sound of the blood pushing its way past is suddenly heard in a stethoscope placed over the artery. This is the maximum pressure reached by the heart during its contraction. As the pressure is further released the sound gradually muffles and disappears the lowest

pressure in your blood system. Putting the two pressures over each other gives a ratio of the blood pressure while the heart is contracting (systolic) over the pressure while the heart is refilling with blood ready for the next contraction (diastolic). The lower pressure actually represents the pressure caused by the major arteries contracting keeping the blood moving while the heart refills.

There is no 'normal' blood pressure as it constantly changes within the same person and depends on what they are doing at the time. A blood pressure of above 140/90 for anyone at rest should be investigated.

Coronary Artery Bypass Graft (CABG)

Introduction

Thanks to this procedure, the outlook for people with blocked coronary arteries has improved dramatically. The coronary artery bypass graft is an effective form of treatment for people with severe coronary artery narrowing from the arterial disease atherosclerosis. The outlook for bypass surgery is best in those who have not had a heart attack and whose hearts are not enlarged and

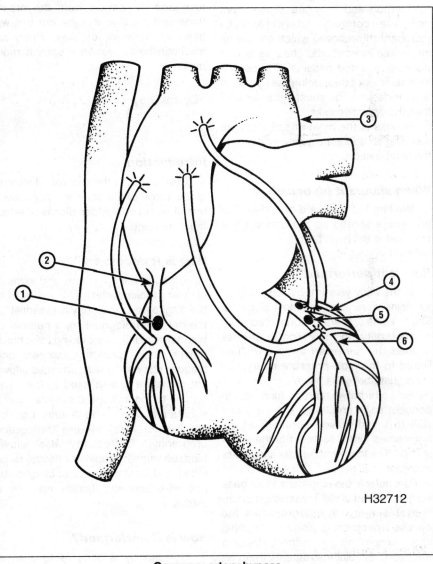

H32712

Coronary artery bypass

1 Blockage	4 Left circumflex artery
2 Right coronary artery	5 Blockage
3 Aorta	6 Left anterior descending artery

there is then an 85% chance of full recovery from all symptoms and a mortality rate, attributable to the operation, of less than two per cent.

The two coronary arteries themselves come off the main artery of the body, the aorta. The left coronary artery immediately divides into two, so there are three main coronary branches. If necessary, a bypass can be done on all three. This is called a triple bypass.

Why is it necessary?

Angina can be not only painful but also debilitating effectively limiting normal life. It can reduce their tolerance to exertion and they are at risk from complete coronary artery blockage (coronary thrombosis) which causes an immediate heart attack. The operation is done on selected patients in whom the long-term risk of not doing the operation is considered to be substantially greater than the operative risks.

Bypass is the most effective way of restoring an adequate supply of blood to the heart muscle.

When should it be done?

Waiting too long is a bad idea. The procedure should be performed while the heart is still healthy.

How is it performed?

In the early years of bypass surgery, leg veins were used in almost all cases. The veins were connected by microsurgery, to the coronary arteries beyond the narrowed areas and then linked to the high-pressure artery, the aorta, just above the heart.

An alternative procedure is to connect an internal artery of the chest wall to the diseased coronary artery. Sometimes just a segment of the artery is used. The long-term results are usually excellent.

The latest development in bypass surgery is minimally invasive coronary bypass surgery. In this procedure the bypass operation is done by keyhole (laparoscopic) surgery without stopping the heart. Special instruments that can be passed though narrow ports are used and the surgeon observes the interior on a video monitor. The method is not suitable for all patients.

Alternatively, metal or plastic devices called stents (small tubes) are being increasingly used to hold coronary arteries open.

Results

Roughly 50% of patients are totally relieved of their symptoms by the operation. Another 40% are considerably improved. 10% are not helped.

Recovery

From the classical operation patients are encouraged to get up within a day or two of the operation. There will be some pain and discomfort from the breast bone and the skin incision but this will pass in a week or two. Recovery from minimally invasive surgery is more rapid.

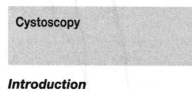

Cystoscopy

Introduction

Cystoscopy is the process of looking at the inside of the bladder – particularly useful as most bladder diseases affect the inner lining.

Why is it necessary?

Although the symptoms and signs of bladder problems can give good clues to the diagnosis, cystoscopy is essential for the definitive diagnosis of a number of bladder conditions including infections, polyps (small growths), cancers and bladder stones. Cystoscopy also allows fine catheters to be passed up the tubes leading to the kidneys (ureters) so that a substance opaque to X-rays can be injected for X-ray studies (retrograde urography). Cystoscopy also allows biopsies (small samples of tissue) to be taken, and local treatment to be given by hot wire cautery, lasers and other means.

How is it performed?

Cystoscopy is done using a small camera called a cystoscope. This is passed in through the urine exit channel (the urethra in the penis). A general anaesthetic is usually required.

In examining the bladder sterile water is run in through a stopcock on the cystoscope. The folds of the bladder flatten out so that the inside of the wall can be inspected. The optical inspection port at the end of the instrument is at an angle, so by rotating the cystoscope the doctor can examine almost the whole of the inside of the bladder.

Hip replacement

Introduction

Hip replacements are now one of the most common surgical procedures in the UK yet it is a relatively recent advance. The actual part of the hip that is replaced is the short neck and rounded ball at the top of the thigh bone, the femur, together with the cup in the side of the pelvis into which the ball of the femur fits to form a ball-and-socket joint.

The hip joint has a wide range of movement and is subject to a range of disorders but those that most commonly call for joint replacement are osteoarthritis, fracture of the neck of the femur, and death of the cells in the head of the femur.

Over 50,000 hip replacements are done every year in Britain.

Because of the smooth, low-friction, connection between the high-density polyethylene socket and the spherical steel or ceramic head, there is no great tendency for the artificial socket to become displaced but, in some cases, loosening has been a problem. The arm of the ball section must be firmly fixed into the hollow shaft of the thigh bone (femur), otherwise this is liable to cause problems in the future.

Why is it necessary?

Waiting too long is not advisable. At the same time all surgery carries a risk so it is a balance. Total hip replacement is necessary when the hip joint has been damaged by arthritis or by loss of its blood supply. Such a hip will be causing considerable pain and disability.

Hip replacement is the only effective treatment for a hip joint that can't function adequately and painlessly.

How is it performed?

The operation is done under an anaesthetic. Hip joint operations are conducted in an ultra-clean environment as any infection which might get inside the bone during the operation is very difficult to treat.

The surgeon cuts off the head of the femur (thigh bone) and clears up the area.

The new cup is now fixed into place using a thick cement. The shaft of thigh bone is cleaned out to remove loose fragments of bone, and the ball is offered up to the new joint. Several positions may have to be tried out.

The results are usually very good but hip replacement is not commonly performed in young and physically active patients.

Rectal examination

Introduction

Nobody pretends that a rectal examination is pleasant or free from embarrassment, but it is an important part of any general examination because it allows the doctor to detect a number of important disorders. Essentially, it involves feeling with a gloved finger, all the structures within reach. The rectum is the short, but distensible, length of bowel immediately above the anal canal. The latter is about 5 cm long, so the rectum is readily accessible to an examining gloved finger.

Why is it necessary?

Rectal examination is essential if the medical history suggests a disorder in the lower abdomen, pelvis, lower rectal or anal region. This is also important if there is any suggestion of enlargement of the prostate gland, which is usually a benign condition, but is sometimes due to cancer. The doctor can often detect enlargement of the prostate gland.

How is it performed?

The patient lies on one side and the doctor uses disposable plastic gloves and a lubricant such as a water based jelly. There is a slight sensation as if the bowels are moving. Doctors perform thousands of rectal examinations and are not in the least embarrassed; obviously it can be different for the patient, but talking the procedure through first can help.

Ultrasound

Description

Few people have not heard of ultrasound. It is widely used as a way of scanning without using any radiation such as X-rays.

In ultrasound scanning, a beam of 'sound' is projected into the body. Whenever it meets a surface between tissues of different density, echoes are created and these return to the scanner. A picture of the inside of the body can be created.

Ultrasound of the intensity and frequency used in scanning is completely harmless. To make sure there is good contact with the device producing the ultrasound waves, a gel is applied to the region to be examined. This can be a bit cold but is also harmless.

Uses of ultrasound

It is useful for examining fluid-filled organs such as the gall bladder, and soft organs, such as the liver, pancreas and kidneys. Gallstones and kidney stones are easily detected. Cirrhosis of the liver, liver cysts, abscesses and tumours can all be shown on a screen.

Echocardiography is a sophisticated method of heart examination using ultrasound which reveals the heart's action in detail in scans taken from different directions. Defects of the heart valves and changes in the walls of the main pumping chambers (ventricles) are shown.

Ultrasound waves cannot easily pass through bone or gas, so it is of less use for parts of the body surrounded by bone, such as the brain and spinal cord. The lungs and the intestines are also unsuitable for ultrasound examination.

Vasectomy ('the snip')

Introduction

Despite its almost universal use there are still myths surrounding vasectomy. It is a simple and permanent method of male sterilisation. It has no effect on your sex drive or ejaculation, but the semen no longer carries sperm, which are reabsorbed in each testicle. Sperm doesn't build up inside the testicles. By law you do not need your partner's permission, but some doctors prefer both partners to agree to the operation after information and counselling and you will have to sign a consent form.

All treatment you get is confidential and free, but NHS waiting lists for sterilisation can be quite long depending on where you live. The operation can also be done privately.

Why should it be done?

It does not interfere with sex or your enjoyment of sex and it is a permanent method of contraception.

When should it be done?

Although it can be performed at any stage of life young, childless men are discouraged as they may regret it later on. You should get full information and counselling if you want to be sterilised. This gives you a chance to talk about the operation in detail and any doubts, worries or questions you might have.

You should not decide to be sterilised if you or your partner are not completely sure or if you are under any stress, for example after a birth, miscarriage, abortion or family or relationship crisis.

How is it performed?

There is now a choice of places to have a vasectomy performed. It is a simple and safe operation lasting around 10-15 minutes, and can be done in a clinic, hospital outpatient department or doctor's surgery. Under a local anaesthetic (it is possible to have a general anaesthetic in some cases), a small section of each vas deferens – the pipes carrying the sperm from the testes – is removed through small cuts on either side of the scrotum. The ends of the tubes are then blocked or stitched. The cuts generally do not need any stitches and heal on their own.

Results

After a vasectomy it usually takes a few months for all the sperm to disappear from your semen. You need to use another method of contraception until you have had **two** consecutive semen tests which show that you have no sperm.

Recovery

There is often some discomfort and swelling lasting for a few days, but this settles quickly with no other problems. Painkillers can help ease the discomfort. Occasionally this can last longer and needs your doctor's attention. Avoid wearing tight underpants and strenuous activity for a week or so.

You can have sex as soon as it is comfortable but at first you will still need to use an extra method of contraception until you have had two clear semen tests.

Your testicles will produce male hormone (testosterone) the same as before your vasectomy. Your feelings, sex drive, ability to have an erection and orgasm won't be affected. The only difference will be that there will not be any sperm in the semen.

There are no known long term risks from a vasectomy.

Future prospects

Even if a vasectomy has been confirmed as a success (after two clear semen tests) about 1 in 2,000 male sterilisations fail. There is a reversal operation but it is not always successful. Not only will the success of your reversal operation depend upon how and when you were sterilised, it is not easily available on the NHS.

Remember that a vasectomy does not protect you against sexually transmitted infections.

If you would like to know more, look in the Contents section at the back of this manual, or contact:

fpa UK,
2-12 Pentonville Road, London, N1 9FP.
Phone 0845 310 1334 (9am to 7pm)
www.fpa.org.uk

Early warning signs — TRADESMAN'S TIPS

When you are driving your car, you have two choices when the oil pressure warning light comes on:
  a) *Stop and put oil in the engine.*
  b) *Rip the light out of the dashboard.*
     Both of these options have the desired effect of no longer seeing a warning light, but only one of them guarantees happy hours finding a reconditioned engine. This is true of many instrument indicators and changes in the behaviour of the car. Few men would continue driving with steam pouring out of the radiator or loose steering, yet we will carry on putting up with many symptoms of early disease much longer than do women. Here are some early warning signs from our expert man mechanics that should not be ignored or you might just find yourself looking for some pretty vital second-hand parts.

a) **Oil pressure warning light:** *High blood pressure has few warning signs. That's why it is called the silent killer (see hypertension). Check your blood pressure at least once a year before you develop blood in your urine, tunnel vision or have a stroke.*

b) **Ignition warning light:** *If you are not charging your battery you will soon not be able to start your engine. Losing weight, a loss of appetite or difficulty in eating needs your doctor's attention (see diabetes and cancer).*

c) **Rev counter:** *If you are over-revving on slight inclines your engine will wear out prematurely. Being unfit is one cause of a high heart rate which refuses to return to normal quickly after exercise (see routine maintenance).*

d) **Speedometer:** *KPH or MPH, if you can't seem to get past idling speed you need to see your doctor or think seriously about some more exercise.*

e) **Brake warning light:** *Not being able to resist one more drink with days off work, poor sleep, bad temper and friction at home is a sign of the brakes needing attention (see routine maintenance).*

f) **Main Beam warning light:** *Are you peering into the gloom? Maybe your eyes need testing. Diabetes is a common cause of eye problems (see diabetes).*

g) **Temperature gauge:** *Over heating is a common sign of obesity. You may find your radiator boiling over as well. This can affect your heart, pancreas and blood vessels, not to mention your erectile function.*

h) **Fuel gauge:** *Trouble with your erections? You may have an underlying condition causing erectile dysfunction or impotence (see erection problems & diabetes).*

j) **Seat belt warning noise:** *Taking unnecessary risks? Young men are much more likely than older men to risk their lives through fast driving, not wearing protective clothing and failing to see their doctor when they find something wrong.*

k) **Low tyre pressure:** *Feeling down? Depression is grossly under-diagnosed in men while suicide is four times higher than in women. Look out for loss of interest, 'short fuses', alcohol abuse, loss of libido or thoughts of harming yourself (see depression).*

l) **High exhaust gas emissions & backfire:** *Inefficient fuel combustion is similar to poor digestion which can result from various problems not least cancer. Blood in your stool is a warning sign not to be ignored.*

m) **Engine misfire:** *Timing is just as important to the heart as it is to the car engine. An irregular heart rate, especially with exercise, needs attention (see atrial fibrillation).*

n) **Engine labouring:** *Pain in the chest could be a sign of problems with your heart (see angina, heart attack).*

p) **Direction indicator failure:** *Bad earth? Poor circulation and nerve disorders can cause problems with the body's 'electrics' (see stroke & diabetes).*

q) **STOP warning indicator:** *Hopefully after reading this section you will never see this indicator come on, or at least not until you can be classified as a vintage model.*

Make no mistake, you are in control of your body but good drivers take heed of warning signs.

Hair Loss (men)

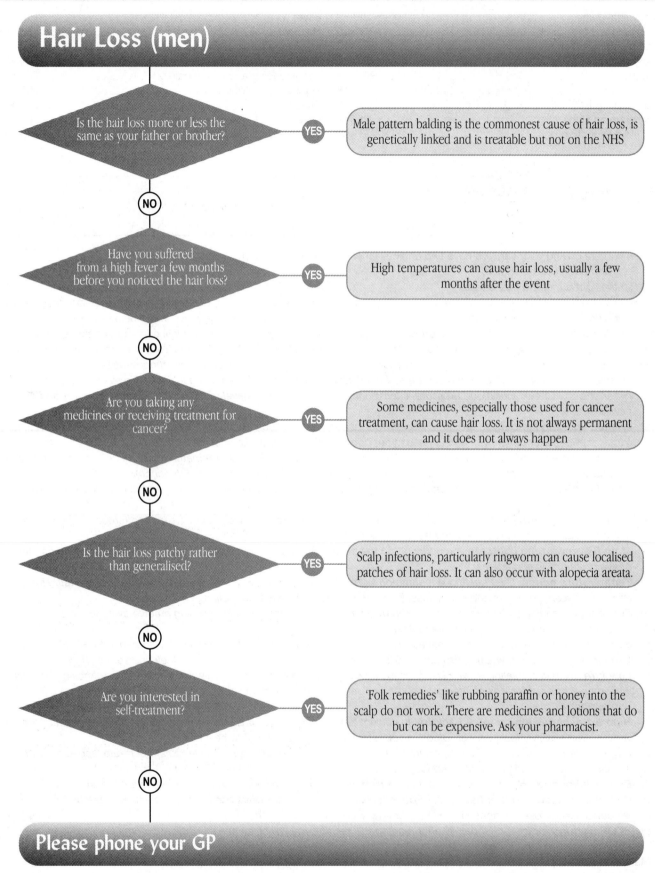

Is the hair loss more or less the same as your father or brother? — **YES** → Male pattern balding is the commonest cause of hair loss, is genetically linked and is treatable but not on the NHS

NO

Have you suffered from a high fever a few months before you noticed the hair loss? — **YES** → High temperatures can cause hair loss, usually a few months after the event

NO

Are you taking any medicines or receiving treatment for cancer? — **YES** → Some medicines, especially those used for cancer treatment, can cause hair loss. It is not always permanent and it does not always happen

NO

Is the hair loss patchy rather than generalised? — **YES** → Scalp infections, particularly ringworm can cause localised patches of hair loss. It can also occur with alopecia areata.

NO

Are you interested in self-treatment? — **YES** → 'Folk remedies' like rubbing paraffin or honey into the scalp do not work. There are medicines and lotions that do but can be expensive. Ask your pharmacist.

NO

Please phone your GP

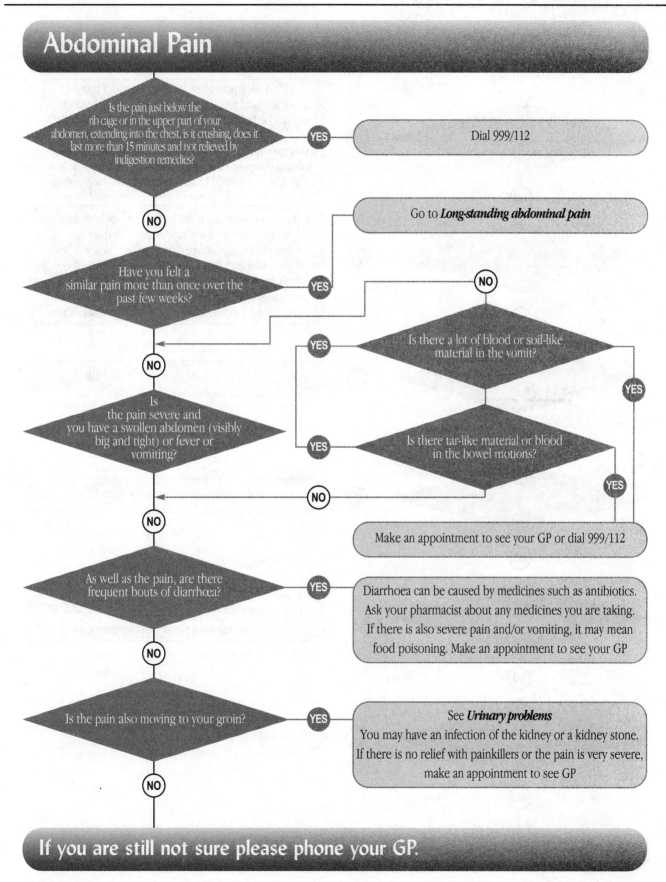

Abdominal Pain

Is the pain just below the rib cage or in the upper part of your abdomen, extending into the chest, is it crushing, does it last more than 15 minutes and not relieved by indigestion remedies? — **YES** → Dial 999/112

NO

Go to *Long-standing abdominal pain*

Have you felt a similar pain more than once over the past few weeks? — **YES**

NO

Is there a lot of blood or soil-like material in the vomit? — **NO** / **YES**

Is the pain severe and you have a swollen abdomen (visibly big and tight) or fever or vomiting? — **YES**

Is there tar-like material or blood in the bowel motions? — **YES**

NO

Make an appointment to see your GP or dial 999/112

NO

As well as the pain, are there frequent bouts of diarrhœa? — **YES** → Diarrhoea can be caused by medicines such as antibiotics. Ask your pharmacist about any medicines you are taking. If there is also severe pain and/or vomiting, it may mean food poisoning. Make an appointment to see your GP

NO

Is the pain also moving to your groin? — **YES** → See *Urinary problems*
You may have an infection of the kidney or a kidney stone. If there is no relief with painkillers or the pain is very severe, make an appointment to see GP

NO

If you are still not sure please phone your GP.

Back Pain

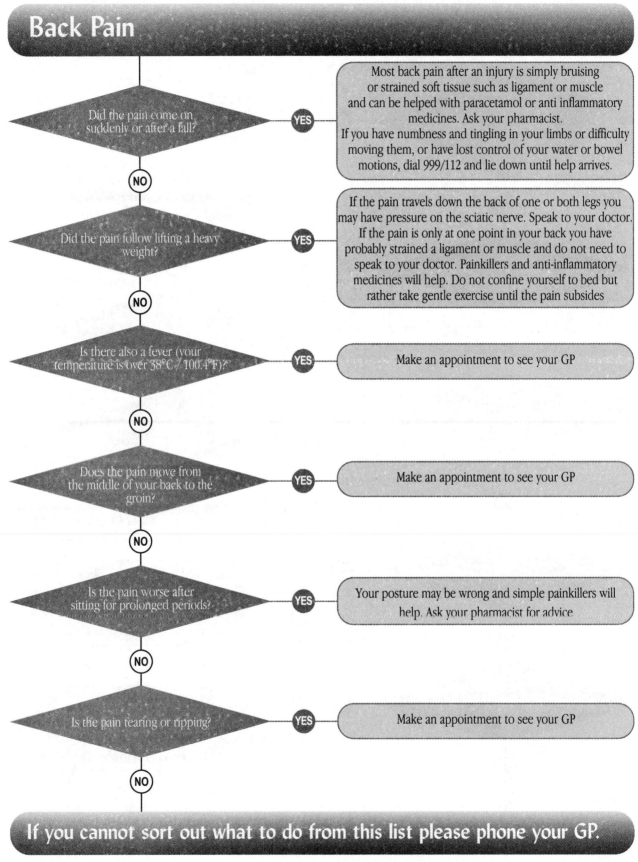

Did the pain come on suddenly or after a fall?

YES → Most back pain after an injury is simply bruising or strained soft tissue such as ligament or muscle and can be helped with paracetamol or anti inflammatory medicines. Ask your pharmacist.
If you have numbness and tingling in your limbs or difficulty moving them, or have lost control of your water or bowel motions, dial 999/112 and lie down until help arrives.

NO

Did the pain follow lifting a heavy weight?

YES → If the pain travels down the back of one or both legs you may have pressure on the sciatic nerve. Speak to your doctor. If the pain is only at one point in your back you have probably strained a ligament or muscle and do not need to speak to your doctor. Painkillers and anti-inflammatory medicines will help. Do not confine yourself to bed but rather take gentle exercise until the pain subsides

NO

Is there also a fever (your temperature is over 38°C / 100.4°F)?

YES → Make an appointment to see your GP

NO

Does the pain move from the middle of your back to the groin?

YES → Make an appointment to see your GP

NO

Is the pain worse after sitting for prolonged periods?

YES → Your posture may be wrong and simple painkillers will help. Ask your pharmacist for advice.

NO

Is the pain tearing or ripping?

YES → Make an appointment to see your GP

NO

If you cannot sort out what to do from this list please phone your GP.

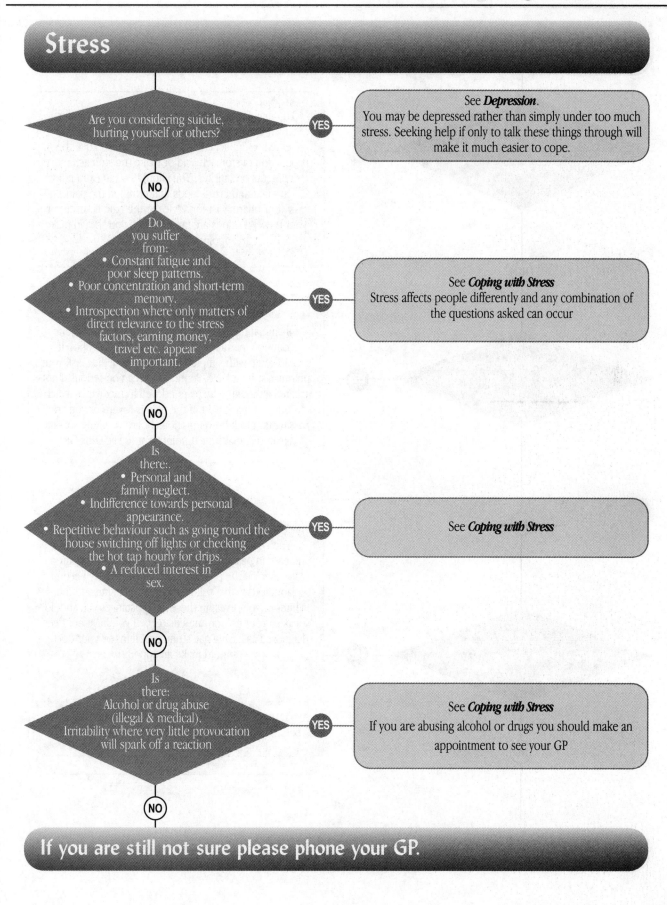

Stress

Are you considering suicide, hurting yourself or others?

YES → See ***Depression***.
You may be depressed rather than simply under too much stress. Seeking help if only to talk these things through will make it much easier to cope.

NO ↓

Do you suffer from:
• Constant fatigue and poor sleep patterns.
• Poor concentration and short-term memory.
• Introspection where only matters of direct relevance to the stress factors, earning money, travel etc. appear important.

YES → See ***Coping with Stress***
Stress affects people differently and any combination of the questions asked can occur

NO ↓

Is there:
• Personal and family neglect.
• Indifference towards personal appearance.
• Repetitive behaviour such as going round the house switching off lights or checking the hot tap hourly for drips.
• A reduced interest in sex.

YES → See ***Coping with Stress***

NO ↓

Is there:
Alcohol or drug abuse (illegal & medical).
Irritability where very little provocation will spark off a reaction

YES → See ***Coping with Stress***
If you are abusing alcohol or drugs you should make an appointment to see your GP

NO ↓

If you are still not sure please phone your GP.

Long-standing abdominal pain

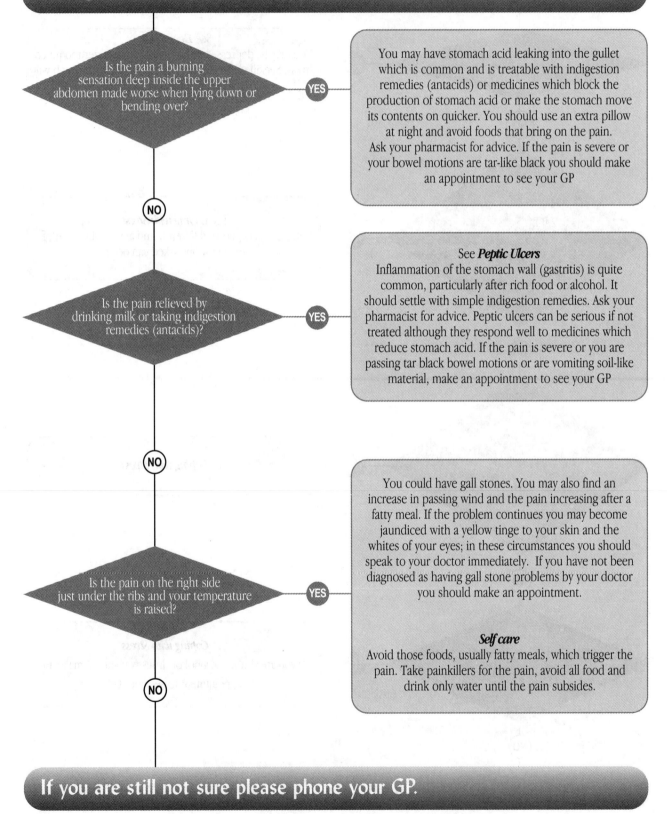

Is the pain a burning sensation deep inside the upper abdomen made worse when lying down or bending over?

YES

You may have stomach acid leaking into the gullet which is common and is treatable with indigestion remedies (antacids) or medicines which block the production of stomach acid or make the stomach move its contents on quicker. You should use an extra pillow at night and avoid foods that bring on the pain. Ask your pharmacist for advice. If the pain is severe or your bowel motions are tar-like black you should make an appointment to see your GP

NO

Is the pain relieved by drinking milk or taking indigestion remedies (antacids)?

YES

See ***Peptic Ulcers***
Inflammation of the stomach wall (gastritis) is quite common, particularly after rich food or alcohol. It should settle with simple indigestion remedies. Ask your pharmacist for advice. Peptic ulcers can be serious if not treated although they respond well to medicines which reduce stomach acid. If the pain is severe or you are passing tar black bowel motions or are vomiting soil-like material, make an appointment to see your GP

NO

Is the pain on the right side just under the ribs and your temperature is raised?

YES

You could have gall stones. You may also find an increase in passing wind and the pain increasing after a fatty meal. If the problem continues you may become jaundiced with a yellow tinge to your skin and the whites of your eyes; in these circumstances you should speak to your doctor immediately. If you have not been diagnosed as having gall stone problems by your doctor you should make an appointment.

Self care
Avoid those foods, usually fatty meals, which trigger the pain. Take painkillers for the pain, avoid all food and drink only water until the pain subsides.

NO

If you are still not sure please phone your GP.

Breathing Difficulty

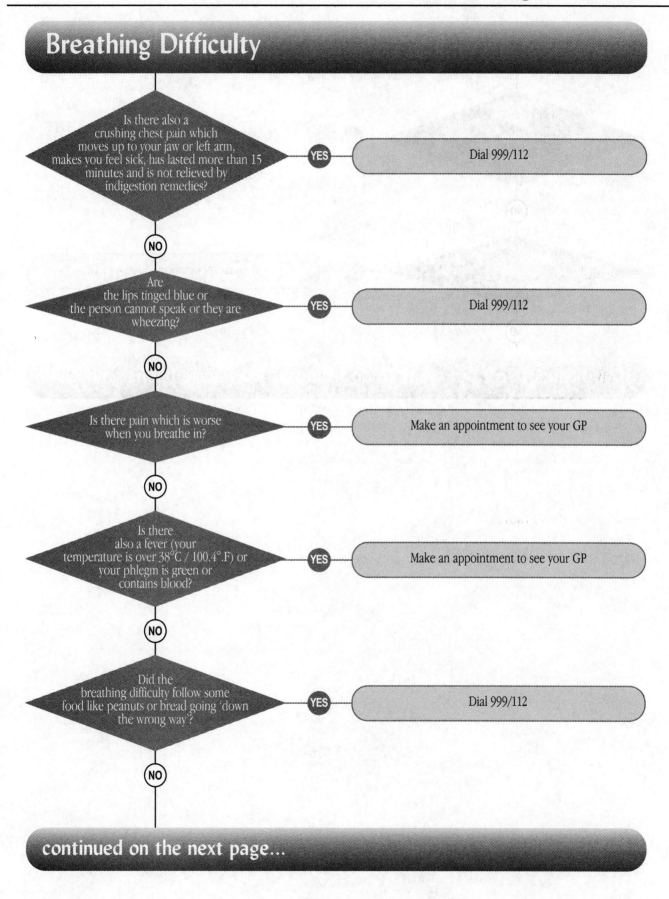

Is there also a crushing chest pain which moves up to your jaw or left arm, makes you feel sick, has lasted more than 15 minutes and is not relieved by indigestion remedies?

YES → Dial 999/112

NO

Are the lips tinged blue or the person cannot speak or they are wheezing?

YES → Dial 999/112

NO

Is there pain which is worse when you breathe in?

YES → Make an appointment to see your GP

NO

Is there also a fever (your temperature is over 38°C / 100.4°.F) or your phlegm is green or contains blood?

YES → Make an appointment to see your GP

NO

Did the breathing difficulty follow some food like peanuts or bread going 'down the wrong way'?

YES → Dial 999/112

NO

continued on the next page...

Breathing Difficulty (continued)

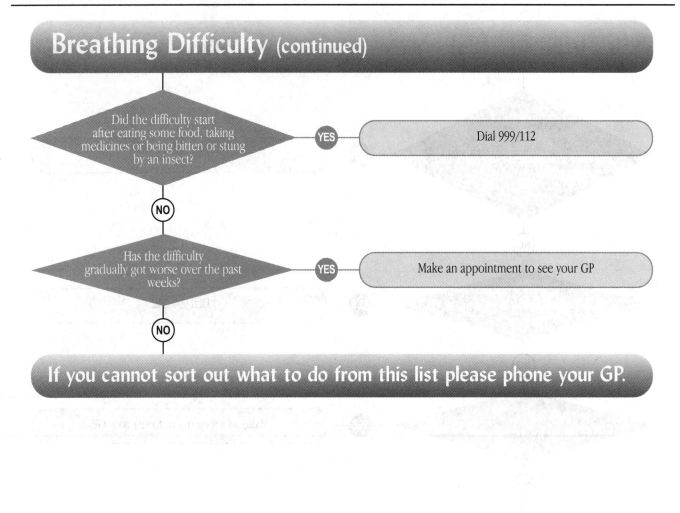

Did the difficulty start after eating some food, taking medicines or being bitten or stung by an insect? — **YES** → Dial 999/112

NO

Has the difficulty gradually got worse over the past weeks? — **YES** → Make an appointment to see your GP

NO

If you cannot sort out what to do from this list please phone your GP.

Chest pain

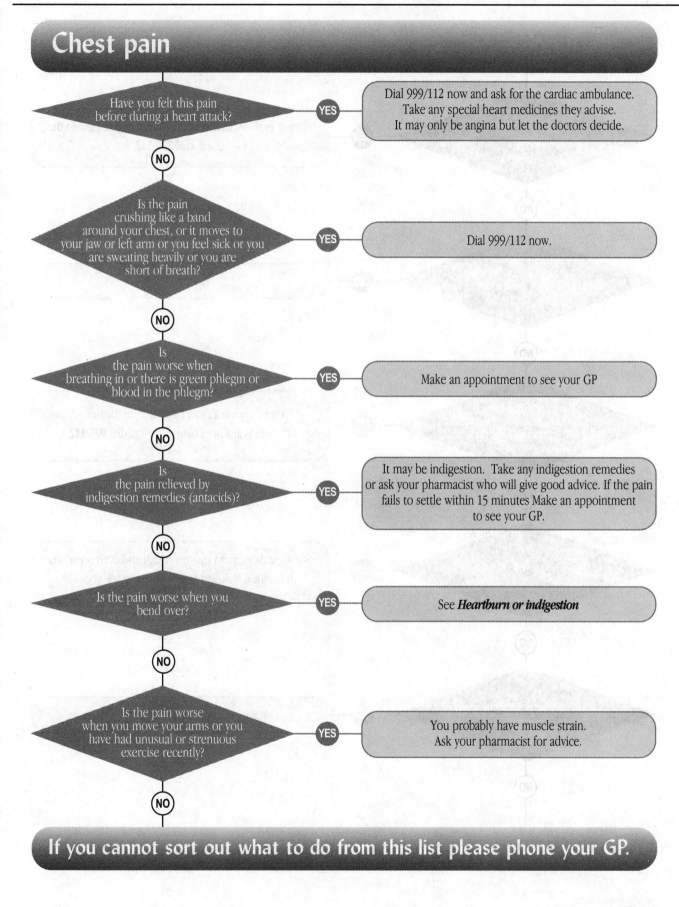

Have you felt this pain before during a heart attack?

YES → Dial 999/112 now and ask for the cardiac ambulance. Take any special heart medicines they advise. It may only be angina but let the doctors decide.

NO

Is the pain crushing like a band around your chest, or it moves to your jaw or left arm or you feel sick or you are sweating heavily or you are short of breath?

YES → Dial 999/112 now.

NO

Is the pain worse when breathing in or there is green phlegm or blood in the phlegm?

YES → Make an appointment to see your GP

NO

Is the pain relieved by indigestion remedies (antacids)?

YES → It may be indigestion. Take any indigestion remedies or ask your pharmacist who will give good advice. If the pain fails to settle within 15 minutes Make an appointment to see your GP.

NO

Is the pain worse when you bend over?

YES → See *Heartburn or indigestion*

NO

Is the pain worse when you move your arms or you have had unusual or strenuous exercise recently?

YES → You probably have muscle strain. Ask your pharmacist for advice.

NO

If you cannot sort out what to do from this list please phone your GP.

Coughing

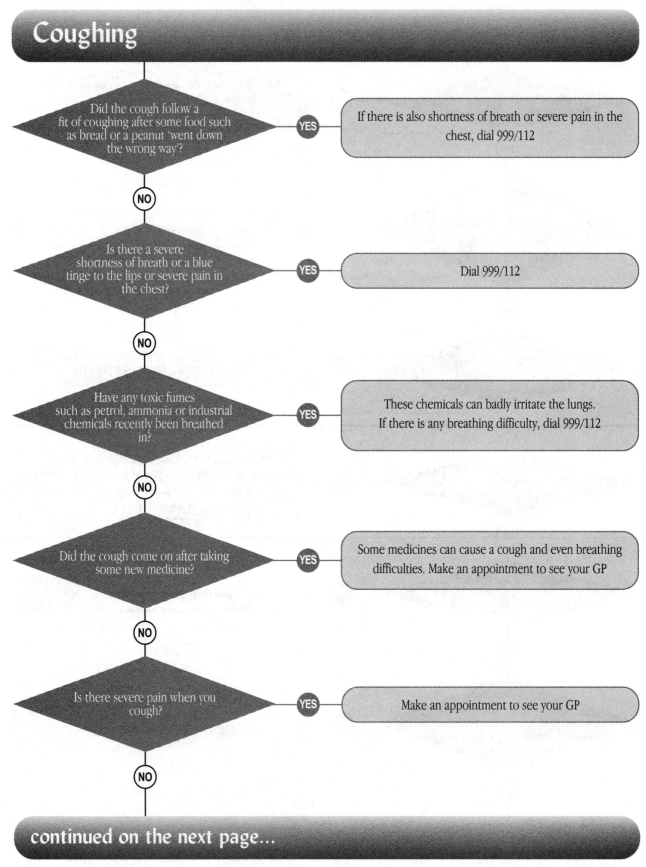

Did the cough follow a fit of coughing after some food such as bread or a peanut 'went down the wrong way'?

YES → If there is also shortness of breath or severe pain in the chest, dial 999/112

NO

Is there a severe shortness of breath or a blue tinge to the lips or severe pain in the chest?

YES → Dial 999/112

NO

Have any toxic fumes such as petrol, ammonia or industrial chemicals recently been breathed in?

YES → These chemicals can badly irritate the lungs. If there is any breathing difficulty, dial 999/112

NO

Did the cough come on after taking some new medicine?

YES → Some medicines can cause a cough and even breathing difficulties. Make an appointment to see your GP

NO

Is there severe pain when you cough?

YES → Make an appointment to see your GP

NO

continued on the next page...

Coughing continued...

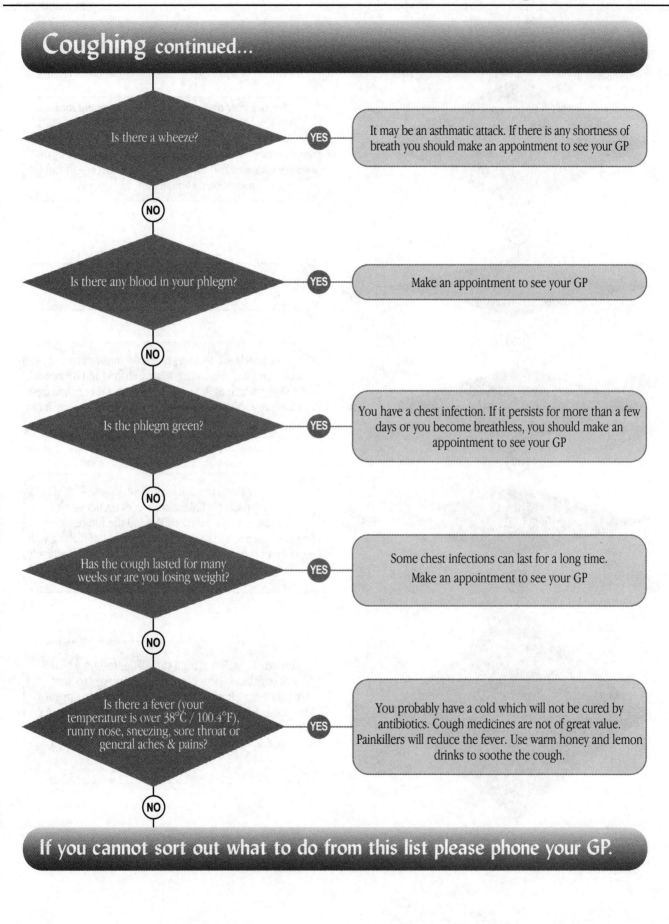

Is there a wheeze? — YES → It may be an asthmatic attack. If there is any shortness of breath you should make an appointment to see your GP

NO

Is there any blood in your phlegm? — YES → Make an appointment to see your GP

NO

Is the phlegm green? — YES → You have a chest infection. If it persists for more than a few days or you become breathless, you should make an appointment to see your GP

NO

Has the cough lasted for many weeks or are you losing weight? — YES → Some chest infections can last for a long time. Make an appointment to see your GP

NO

Is there a fever (your temperature is over 38°C / 100.4°F), runny nose, sneezing, sore throat or general aches & pains? — YES → You probably have a cold which will not be cured by antibiotics. Cough medicines are not of great value. Painkillers will reduce the fever. Use warm honey and lemon drinks to soothe the cough.

NO

If you cannot sort out what to do from this list please phone your GP.

Depression

Did any of the feelings of despair, sadness, grief, unworthiness, guilt or inability to cope come after serious life events such as a bereavement, splitting up with a partner or losing your job?

YES → See *Grieving and coping with bereavement and Relaxation exercises*
This kind of depression is normal but nonetheless a terrible experience. Tranquillisers are not a good idea. Activity that takes your mind off the reason for your depression and relaxation techniques are far better

NO ↓

Are you taking any medicines at present?

YES → Some medicines can affect your mood especially if mixed with alcohol

NO ↓

Are you recovering after a viral illness such as glandular fever, flu or hepatitis?

YES → Some infectious diseases, especially those caused by viruses, can leave you feeling weak, lethargic and depressed. (post viral syndrome). Keeping active with a diet rich in fresh fruit and vegetables helps but there is no medical cure. It can last from weeks to months.

NO ↓

Has your partner recently given birth?

YES → Male post natal depression exists.
It is probably linked to a mix of tiredness, anxiety over relationships and the future.
Remaining active and using relaxation techniques along with good support from partners, friends and family undoubtedly helps but rarely some men may need medical help.

NO ↓

Are you experiencing for no apparent reason:
- A crushing despair?
- Disturbed sleep with early waking?
- Noticeable and unintended weight changes?
- Alcohol abuse?
- Lost of interest in work or family?
- Inability to concentrate on a job?
- Withdrawal from family or friends?
- A feeling of low self esteem?
- General fatigue?
- Thoughts of suicide?

YES → You may be suffering from clinical depression which is not made any better by people telling you to 'sort yourself out'. It is best helped with medical treatment. You should see your doctor especially if you are having thoughts of suicide. There are many things that can be done to help you and you do not need to suffer in silence.

If you are still not sure please phone your GP.

Diarrhoea

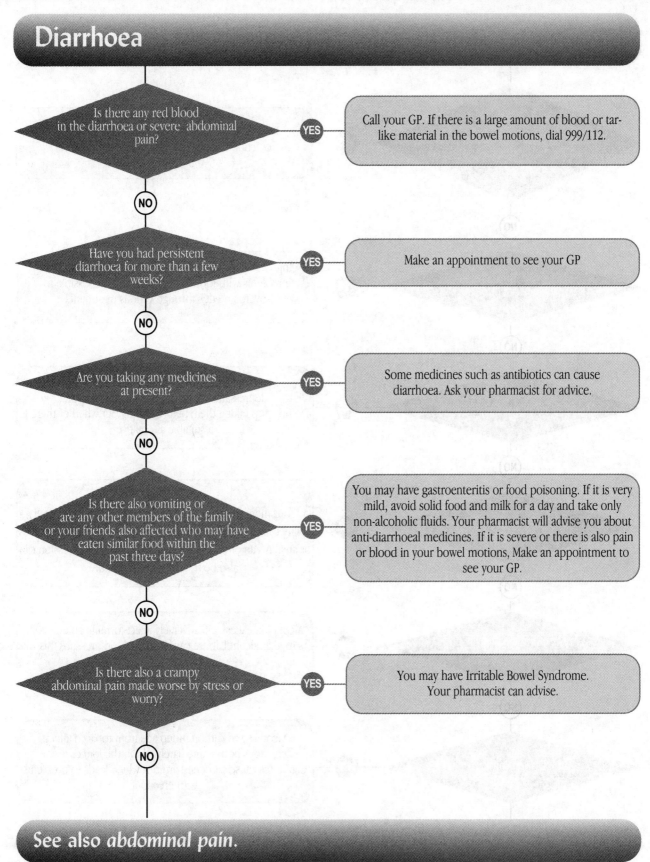

Is there any red blood in the diarrhoea or severe abdominal pain?

YES → Call your GP. If there is a large amount of blood or tar-like material in the bowel motions, dial 999/112.

NO

Have you had persistent diarrhoea for more than a few weeks?

YES → Make an appointment to see your GP

NO

Are you taking any medicines at present?

YES → Some medicines such as antibiotics can cause diarrhoea. Ask your pharmacist for advice.

NO

Is there also vomiting or are any other members of the family or your friends also affected who may have eaten similar food within the past three days?

YES → You may have gastroenteritis or food poisoning. If it is very mild, avoid solid food and milk for a day and take only non-alcoholic fluids. Your pharmacist will advise you about anti-diarrhoeal medicines. If it is severe or there is also pain or blood in your bowel motions, Make an appointment to see your GP.

NO

Is there also a crampy abdominal pain made worse by stress or worry?

YES → You may have Irritable Bowel Syndrome. Your pharmacist can advise.

NO

See also *abdominal pain.*

Erectile Dysfunction (Impotence)

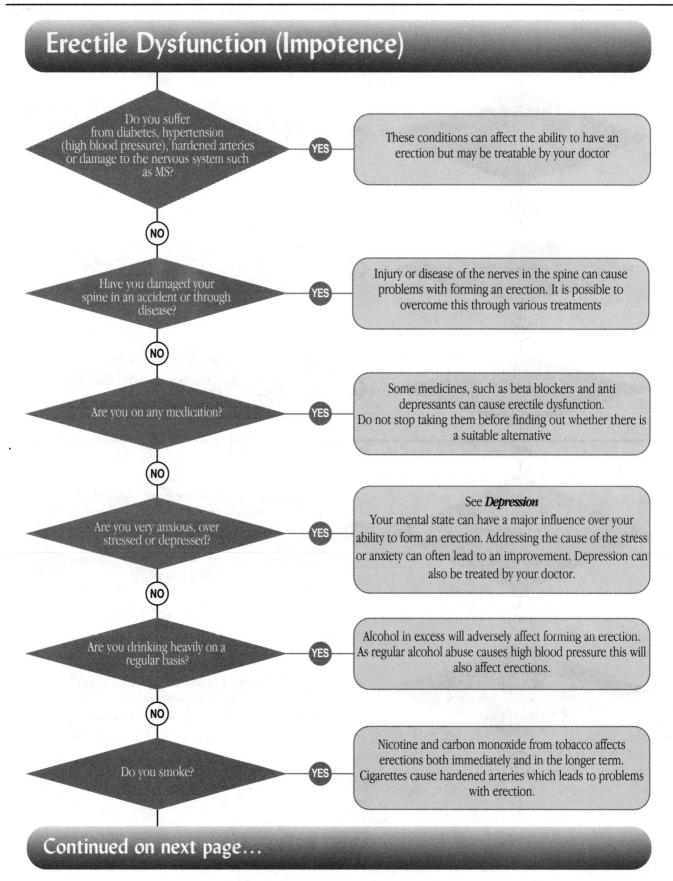

Do you suffer from diabetes, hypertension (high blood pressure), hardened arteries or damage to the nervous system such as MS?

YES — These conditions can affect the ability to have an erection but may be treatable by your doctor

NO

Have you damaged your spine in an accident or through disease?

YES — Injury or disease of the nerves in the spine can cause problems with forming an erection. It is possible to overcome this through various treatments

NO

Are you on any medication?

YES — Some medicines, such as beta blockers and anti depressants can cause erectile dysfunction. Do not stop taking them before finding out whether there is a suitable alternative

NO

Are you very anxious, over stressed or depressed?

YES — See *Depression*
Your mental state can have a major influence over your ability to form an erection. Addressing the cause of the stress or anxiety can often lead to an improvement. Depression can also be treated by your doctor.

NO

Are you drinking heavily on a regular basis?

YES — Alcohol in excess will adversely affect forming an erection. As regular alcohol abuse causes high blood pressure this will also affect erections.

NO

Do you smoke?

YES — Nicotine and carbon monoxide from tobacco affects erections both immediately and in the longer term. Cigarettes cause hardened arteries which leads to problems with erection.

Continued on next page...

Erectile Dysfunction (Impotence) continued...

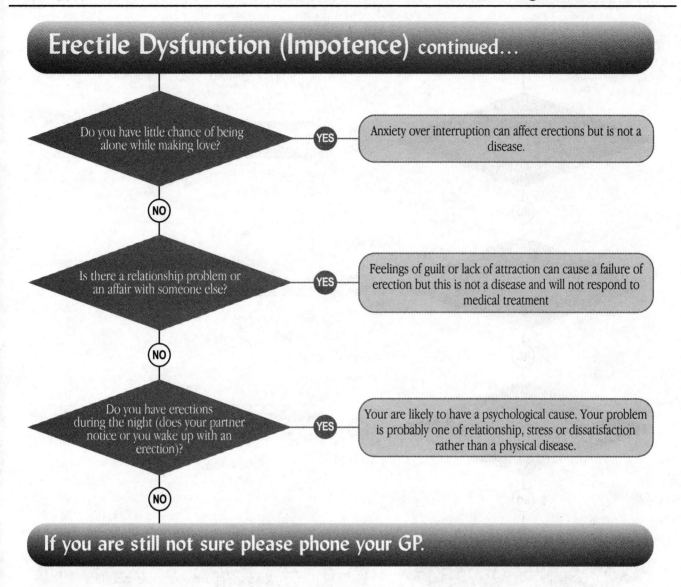

Do you have little chance of being alone while making love?

YES → Anxiety over interruption can affect erections but is not a disease.

NO

Is there a relationship problem or an affair with someone else?

YES → Feelings of guilt or lack of attraction can cause a failure of erection but this is not a disease and will not respond to medical treatment

NO

Do you have erections during the night (does your partner notice or you wake up with an erection)?

YES → Your are likely to have a psychological cause. Your problem is probably one of relationship, stress or dissatisfaction rather than a physical disease.

NO

If you are still not sure please phone your GP.

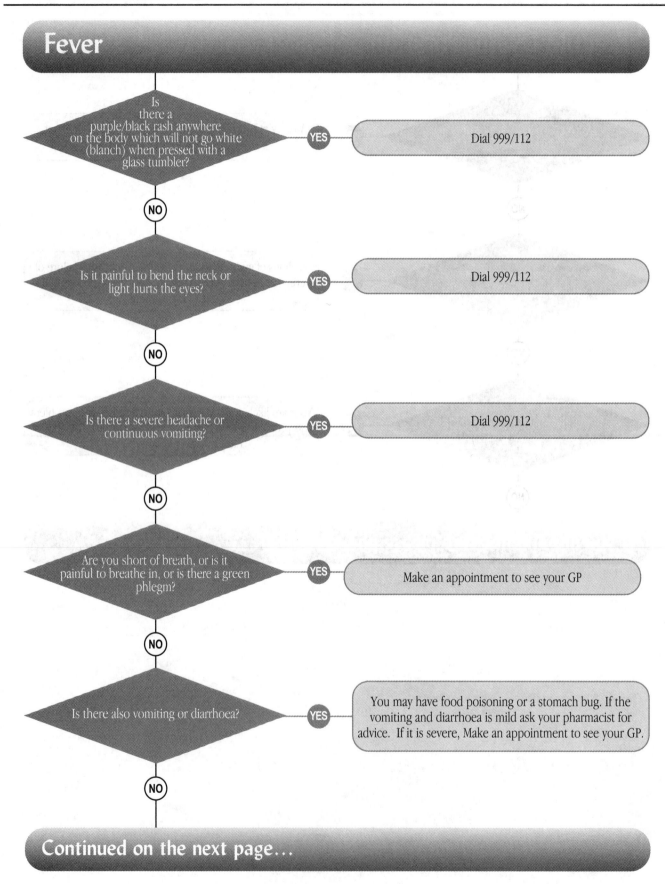

Fever

Is there a purple/black rash anywhere on the body which will not go white (blanch) when pressed with a glass tumbler? — **YES** → Dial 999/112

NO ↓

Is it painful to bend the neck or light hurts the eyes? — **YES** → Dial 999/112

NO ↓

Is there a severe headache or continuous vomiting? — **YES** → Dial 999/112

NO ↓

Are you short of breath, or is it painful to breathe in, or is there a green phlegm? — **YES** → Make an appointment to see your GP

NO ↓

Is there also vomiting or diarrhoea? — **YES** → You may have food poisoning or a stomach bug. If the vomiting and diarrhoea is mild ask your pharmacist for advice. If it is severe, Make an appointment to see your GP.

NO ↓

Continued on the next page...

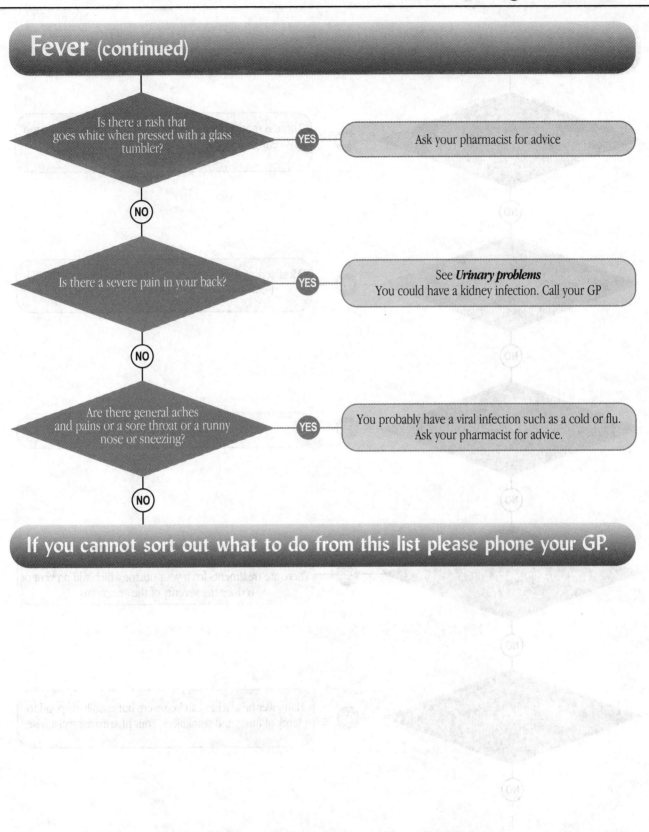

Fever (continued)

Is there a rash that goes white when pressed with a glass tumbler?
— **YES** → Ask your pharmacist for advice

NO

Is there a severe pain in your back?
— **YES** → See *Urinary problems*
You could have a kidney infection. Call your GP

NO

Are there general aches and pains or a sore throat or a runny nose or sneezing?
— **YES** → You probably have a viral infection such as a cold or flu. Ask your pharmacist for advice.

NO

If you cannot sort out what to do from this list please phone your GP.

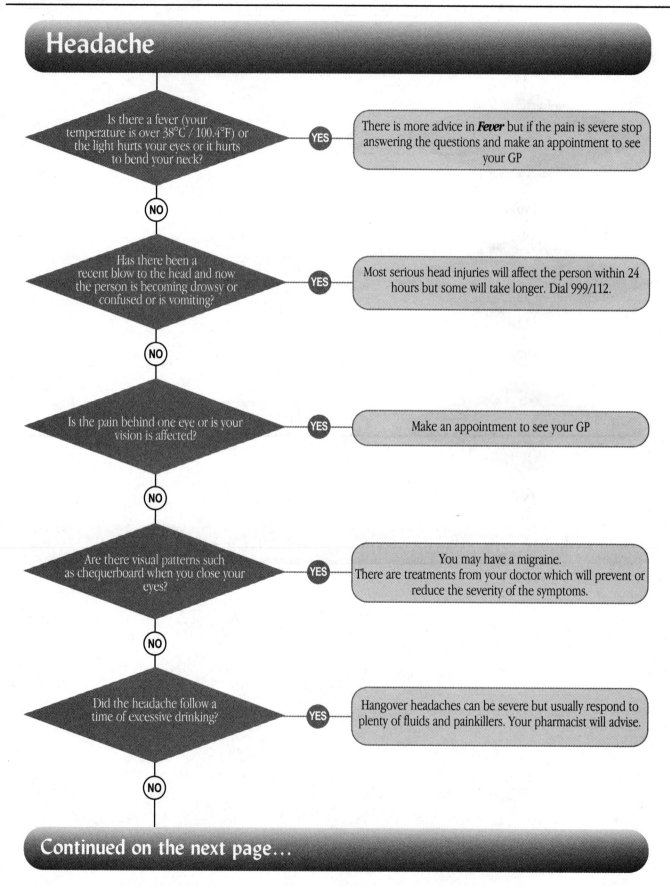

Headache

Is there a fever (your temperature is over 38°C / 100.4°F) or the light hurts your eyes or it hurts to bend your neck?

YES → There is more advice in *Fever* but if the pain is severe stop answering the questions and make an appointment to see your GP

NO ↓

Has there been a recent blow to the head and now the person is becoming drowsy or confused or is vomiting?

YES → Most serious head injuries will affect the person within 24 hours but some will take longer. Dial 999/112.

NO ↓

Is the pain behind one eye or is your vision is affected?

YES → Make an appointment to see your GP

NO ↓

Are there visual patterns such as chequerboard when you close your eyes?

YES → You may have a migraine. There are treatments from your doctor which will prevent or reduce the severity of the symptoms.

NO ↓

Did the headache follow a time of excessive drinking?

YES → Hangover headaches can be severe but usually respond to plenty of fluids and painkillers. Your pharmacist will advise.

NO ↓

Continued on the next page...

Headache (continued)

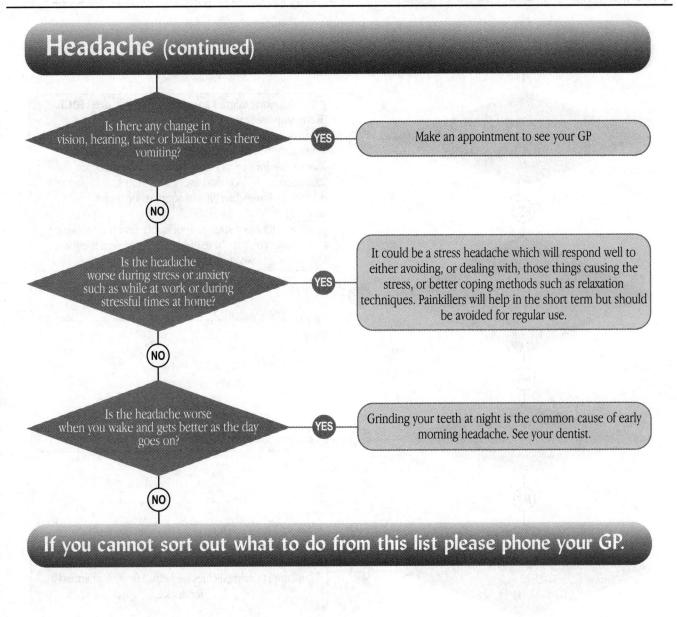

Is there any change in vision, hearing, taste or balance or is there vomiting?

YES → Make an appointment to see your GP

NO

Is the headache worse during stress or anxiety such as while at work or during stressful times at home?

YES → It could be a stress headache which will respond well to either avoiding, or dealing with, those things causing the stress, or better coping methods such as relaxation techniques. Painkillers will help in the short term but should be avoided for regular use.

NO

Is the headache worse when you wake and gets better as the day goes on?

YES → Grinding your teeth at night is the common cause of early morning headache. See your dentist.

NO

If you cannot sort out what to do from this list please phone your GP.

Joint Pain

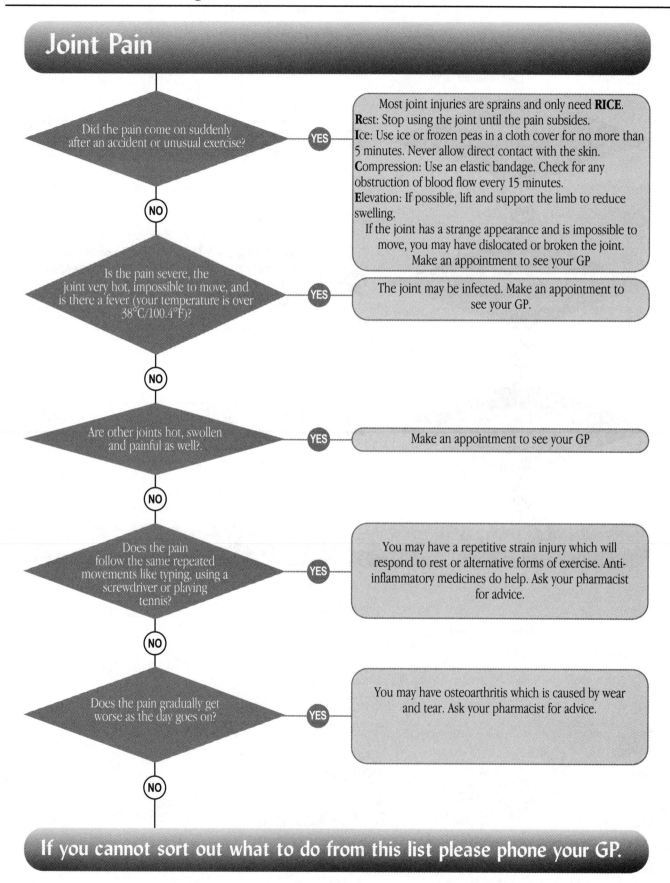

Did the pain come on suddenly after an accident or unusual exercise?

YES → Most joint injuries are sprains and only need **RICE**.
Rest: Stop using the joint until the pain subsides.
Ice: Use ice or frozen peas in a cloth cover for no more than 5 minutes. Never allow direct contact with the skin.
Compression: Use an elastic bandage. Check for any obstruction of blood flow every 15 minutes.
Elevation: If possible, lift and support the limb to reduce swelling.
If the joint has a strange appearance and is impossible to move, you may have dislocated or broken the joint. Make an appointment to see your GP

NO ↓

Is the pain severe, the joint very hot, impossible to move, and is there a fever (your temperature is over 38°C/100.4°F)?

YES → The joint may be infected. Make an appointment to see your GP.

NO ↓

Are other joints hot, swollen and painful as well?.

YES → Make an appointment to see your GP

NO ↓

Does the pain follow the same repeated movements like typing, using a screwdriver or playing tennis?

YES → You may have a repetitive strain injury which will respond to rest or alternative forms of exercise. Anti-inflammatory medicines do help. Ask your pharmacist for advice.

NO ↓

Does the pain gradually get worse as the day goes on?

YES → You may have osteoarthritis which is caused by wear and tear. Ask your pharmacist for advice.

NO ↓

If you cannot sort out what to do from this list please phone your GP.

Tight Foreskin (Phimosis)

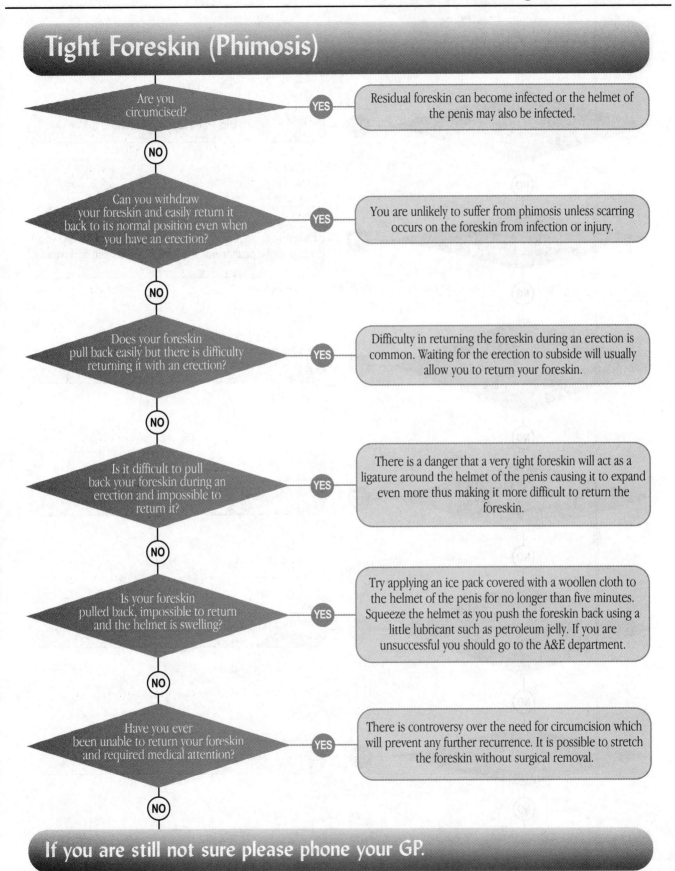

Are you circumcised? — YES → Residual foreskin can become infected or the helmet of the penis may also be infected.

NO ↓

Can you withdraw your foreskin and easily return it back to its normal position even when you have an erection? — YES → You are unlikely to suffer from phimosis unless scarring occurs on the foreskin from infection or injury.

NO ↓

Does your foreskin pull back easily but there is difficulty returning it with an erection? — YES → Difficulty in returning the foreskin during an erection is common. Waiting for the erection to subside will usually allow you to return your foreskin.

NO ↓

Is it difficult to pull back your foreskin during an erection and impossible to return it? — YES → There is a danger that a very tight foreskin will act as a ligature around the helmet of the penis causing it to expand even more thus making it more difficult to return the foreskin.

NO ↓

Is your foreskin pulled back, impossible to return and the helmet is swelling? — YES → Try applying an ice pack covered with a woollen cloth to the helmet of the penis for no longer than five minutes. Squeeze the helmet as you push the foreskin back using a little lubricant such as petroleum jelly. If you are unsuccessful you should go to the A&E department.

NO ↓

Have you ever been unable to return your foreskin and required medical attention? — YES → There is controversy over the need for circumcision which will prevent any further recurrence. It is possible to stretch the foreskin without surgical removal.

NO ↓

If you are still not sure please phone your GP.

Urinary Problems

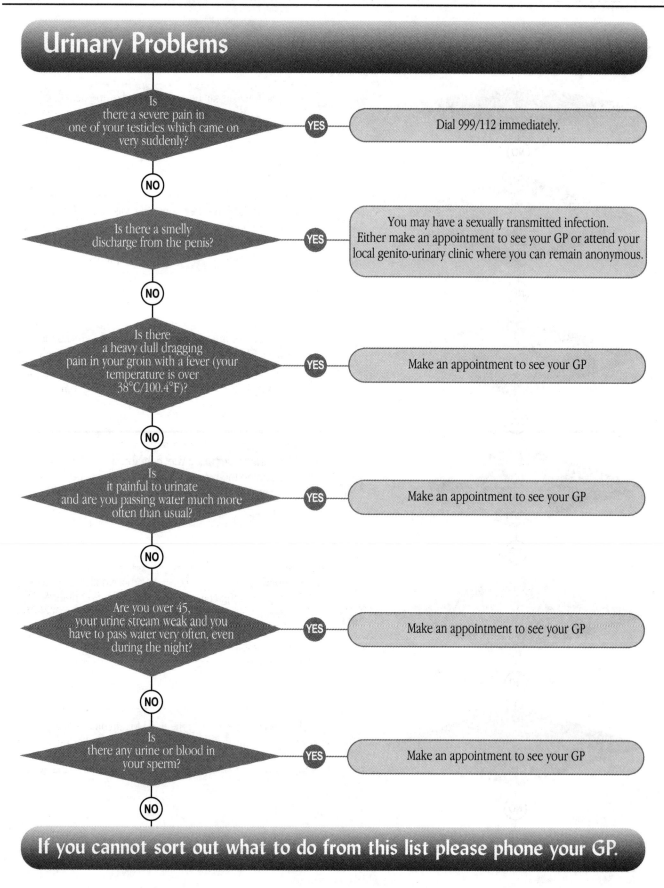

Is there a severe pain in one of your testicles which came on very suddenly? — **YES** → Dial 999/112 immediately.

NO

Is there a smelly discharge from the penis? — **YES** → You may have a sexually transmitted infection. Either make an appointment to see your GP or attend your local genito-urinary clinic where you can remain anonymous.

NO

Is there a heavy dull dragging pain in your groin with a fever (your temperature is over 38°C/100.4°F)? — **YES** → Make an appointment to see your GP

NO

Is it painful to urinate and are you passing water much more often than usual? — **YES** → Make an appointment to see your GP

NO

Are you over 45, your urine stream weak and you have to pass water very often, even during the night? — **YES** → Make an appointment to see your GP

NO

Is there any urine or blood in your sperm? — **YES** → Make an appointment to see your GP

NO

If you cannot sort out what to do from this list please phone your GP.

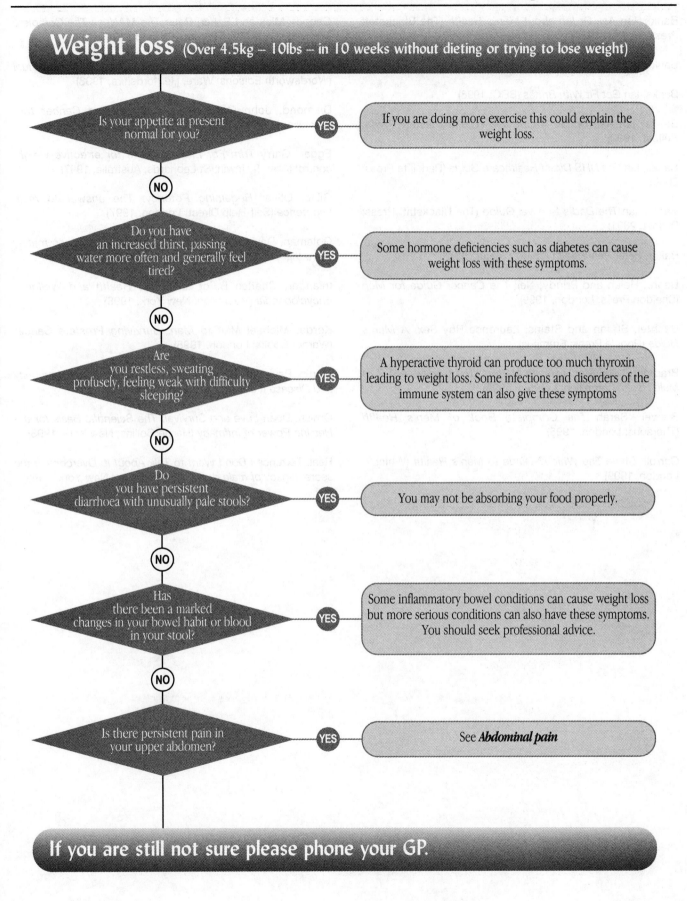

Weight loss (Over 4.5kg – 10lbs – in 10 weeks without dieting or trying to lose weight)

Is your appetite at present normal for you? — YES → If you are doing more exercise this could explain the weight loss.

NO ↓

Do you have an increased thirst, passing water more often and generally feel tired? — YES → Some hormone deficiencies such as diabetes can cause weight loss with these symptoms.

NO ↓

Are you restless, sweating profusely, feeling weak with difficulty sleeping? — YES → A hyperactive thyroid can produce too much thyroxin leading to weight loss. Some infections and disorders of the immune system can also give these symptoms

NO ↓

Do you have persistent diarrhoea with unusually pale stools? — YES → You may not be absorbing your food properly.

NO ↓

Has there been a marked changes in your bowel habit or blood in your stool? — YES → Some inflammatory bowel conditions can cause weight loss but more serious conditions can also have these symptoms. You should seek professional advice.

NO ↓

Is there persistent pain in your upper abdomen? — YES → See *Abdominal pain*

If you are still not sure please phone your GP.

Banks, Ian *Ask Dr Ian about Men's Health* (The Blackstaff Press; Belfast, 1997)

Banks, Ian *The Trouble With Men* (BBC; 1997)

Banks, Ian *Get Fit With Brittas* (BBC; 1998)

Banks, Ian *Ask Dr Ian About Sex* (The Blackstaff Press; Belfast, 1999)

Banks, Ian *The NHS Direct Healthcare Guide* (Radcliffe Press; 2000)

Banks, Ian *The Dad's Survival Guide* (The Blackstaff Press; Belfast, 2001)

Baker, Peter *Real Health for Men* (Vega; 2002)

Beare, Helen and Priddy, Neil *The Cancer Guide for Men* (Sheldon Press; London, 1999)

Bechtel, Stefan and Stains, Laurence Roy *Sex: A Man's Guide* (Rodale Press; Emmaus)

Bradford, Nikki *Men's Health Matters: The Complete A-Z of Male Health* (Vermilion; London, 1995)

Brewer, Sarah *The Complete Book of Men's Health* (Thorsons; London, 1995)

Carroll, Steve *The Which? Guide to Men's Health* (Which?; London, 1999)

Cooper, Mick and Baker, Peter *The MANual: The Complete Man's Guide to Life* (Thorsons; London, 1996)

Diagram Group, The *Man's Body: An Owner's Manual* (Wordsworth Editions; Ware, Hertfordshire, 1998)

Diamond, John *C: Because Cowards get Cancer too.* (Vermilion; London, 1999)

Egger, Garry *Trim For Life: 201 tips for effective weight control* (Allen & Unwin; St Leonards, Australia, 1997)

Gillie, Oliver *Regaining Potency: The answer to male impotence* (Self-Help Direct; London, 1997)

Goleman, Daniel *Emotional Intelligence: Why it can matter more than 10* (Bloomsbury; London, 1996)

Inlander, Charles B. et al. *Men's Health and Wellness Encyclopaedia* (Macmillan; New York, 1998)

Korda, Michael *Man to Man: Surviving Prostate Cancer* (Warner Books; London, 1998).

Martin, Paul *The Sickening Mind: Brain, Behaviour, Immunity and Disease* (Flamingo; London, 1997)

Ornish, Dean *Love and Survival: The Scientific Basis for the Healing Power of Intimacy* (HarperCollins; New York, 1998)

Real, Terrence *I Don't Want to Talk About It: Overcoming the secret legacy of male depression* (Fireside; New York, 1998)

General

Alcoholics Anonymous
PO Box 1
Stonebow House, Stonebow
York YO1 7NJ
Tel: 01904 644026

British Heart Foundation
14 Fitzhardinge Street,
London W1H 6DH
020 7935 0185
www.bhf.org.uk

Diabetes UK
10 Parkway,
London,
NW1 7AA.
Tel: 020 7424 1030

Drinkline
(For advice and information on reducing
alcohol consumption)
Tel: 0800 917 8282

Family Planning Association
(For advice and information on
contraception, sexually transmitted
infections and other sexual health
issues)
2-12 Pentonville Road,
London
N1 9FP
Tel: 0845 310 1334 (mon-fri 9am-7pm)
or 020 7837 4044 5
www.fpa.org.uk

Impotence Association
(For information and advice on all sexual
dysfunctions)
PO Box 10296,
London SW17 9WH
Tel: 020 8767 7791
www.impotence.org.uk

International Stress Management
Association
The Priory Hospital,
Priory Lane,
London,
SW15 5JJ.

MIND (National Association For Mental
Health)
Granta House,
15-19 Broadway,
Stratford,
London,
E15 4BQ.

National Asthma Campaign
Providence House
Providence Place
London N1 0NT
Tel: 020 7226 2260
Fax: 020 7704 0740
www.asthma.org.uk

National Osteoporosis Society
Tel: 01761 471771
www.nos.org.uk

NHS Direct
An online health information service
(includes child health)
Tel: 0845 4647
www.nhsdirect.nhs.uk

Prostate Help Association
Langworth, Lincoln, LN3 5DF

Prostate Research Campaign UK
PO Box 2371,
Swindon, SN1 3LS
Tel 01793 431 901
www.prostate-research.org.uk

QUIT
Ground Floor,
211 Old Street, London EC1V 9NR
Smokers' Quit-line: 0800 00 22 00
www.quit.org.uk

Rethink (previously the NSF)
Head Office,
30 Tabernacle Street,
London, EC2A 4DD.
Tel: 020 7330 9100
www.rethink.org

Samaritans
(For emotional support for people in
crisis or at risk of suicide)
General Office,
10 The Grove,
Slough, Berks, SL1 1QP.
Tel: 08457 90 90 90
www.samaritans.org

St John Ambulance
27 St. John's Lane,
London, EC1M 4BU.
0870-010 4950
www.sja.org.uk

Stroke Association,
Stroke House,
Whitecross Street, London, EC1Y 8JJ.
Tel: 0845 30 33 100

The Prostate Cancer Charity
3 Angel Walk,
Hammersmith,
London W6 9HX.
Tel 0845 300 8383
www.prostate-cancer.org.uk

The Terrence Higgins Trust
(For advice and information on HIV and
AIDS)
52-54 Grays Inn Road,
London WC1X 8JU
020 7242 1010
www.tht.org.uk

World Cancer Research Fund
19 Harley Street,
London, W1G 9QJ.
Tel: 020 7343 4200
Web: www.wcrf-uk.org

FATHERHOOD

Association for Post-Natal Illness
(Provides advice, information and
support mainly to mothers but also runs
a support service for partners)
145 Dawes Road,
Fulham, London SW6 7EB
020 7386 0868
www.apni.org

The Baby Directory
(A commercial site which includes
information on aspects of parenting,
including medical advice and new books
for children and their parents)
www.babydirectory.com

The Baby Registry
(An information site for parents with
some specific sections for dads.)
www.thebabyregistry.co.uk

Babyworld
(A comprehensive commercial site from
Freeserve which contains some specific
sections for dads)
www.babyworld.co.uk

Child Support Agency
(The CSA is the government agency that
ensures that non-resident parents
contribute towards the financial support
of their children)
08457 133 133
www.csa.gov.uk

Dads and Daughters
(A US-based organisation which aims to strengthen men's relationships with their daughters and transform the pervasive messages that value daughters more for how they look than who they are)
www.dadsanddaughters.org

divorce.co.uk
(Advice on mediation, counselling and the legal aspects of divorce from a firm of solicitors)
www.divorce.co.uk

Donor Conception Network.
(For advice, information and support on donor insemination)
PO Box 265, Sheffield S3 7YX.
Tel: 0208 245 4369
www.dcnetwork.org

Families Need Fathers
(Provides legal advice and information mainly about access to children following divorce or separation)
www.fnf.org.uk

Fathers Network
(A US-based organisations that supports fathers and families raising children with special health care needs and developmental disabilities)
www.fathersnetwork.org

The Foundation for the Study of Infant Deaths
(For advice and information on preventing cot death and support following a bereavement)
Artillery House
11-19 Artillery Row, London SW1P 1RT
Tel: 020 7233 2090
www.sids.org.uk/fsid

Gingerbread
Tel: 0800 018 4318
www.gingerbread.org.uk/groups.html

ISSUE: The National Fertility Association
(Provides advice, information and support on fertility problems.)
114 Lichfield Street
Walsall, West Midlands WS1 1SZ
Tel: 01922 722888
www.issue.co.uk

Miscarriage Association
(For advice, information and support about miscarriage)
c/o Clayton Hospital
Northgate, Wakefield
West Yorkshire WF1 3JS
Tel: 01924 200799
www.miscarriageassociation.org.uk

National Center for Fathering
(Provides advice and information for dads - US-based)
www.fathers.com

National Childbirth Trust
(For information on ante-natal classes, childbirth and local groups for parents/fathers)
Alexandra House, Oldham Terrace
London W3 6NH
Tel: 0870 444 8707
www.nct-online.org

National Council for One Parent Families
(Founded in 1918, a national charity working to promote the interests of lone parents and their children and at the forefront of change to improve their lives)
255 Kentish Town Road
London NW5 2LX
Tel: 0800 018 5026
www.oneparentfamilies.org.uk

National Fatherhood Initiative
(US-based non-profit, non-sectarian, non-partisan organisation that promotes responsible fatherhood)
www.fatherhood.org

New dads
(A US organisation that provides information for new fathers)
www.newdads.com

New Ways To Work
(Provides information and advice on flexible working arrangements)
Tel: 0207 503 3578
www.new-ways.co.uk

Parentline plus
(Runs a confidential freephone helpline for all parents. Also provides training courses for parents and written information)
0808 800 2222
Mon-Fri 9am-9pm, Sat 9.30am-5pm, Sun10am-3pm.
Textphone/minicom: 0800 783 6783.
email: headoffice@parentlineplus.org.uk
www.parentlineplus.org.uk

Parents at Work
(For information on parents' employment rights)
45 Beech Street
London EC2Y 8AD
Tel: 0207 628 3578
www.parentsatwork.org.uk

Parents Online
(Provides information to help parents with children through their primary school years)
www.parents.org.uk

Relate
(For counselling for relationship and/or sexual problems)
Tel: 0845 1304010
www.relate.org.uk

Serene
(An advice and information service for parents of excessively crying, sleepless and demanding babies and young children)
Tel: 020 7404 5011
www.our-space.co.uk/serene.htm

Sex Education Forum
(Provides information and guidance to parents)
Tel: 020 7843 6052
www.ncb.org.uk/sef/index.htm

Shared Parenting Information Group (SPIG) UK
(An organisation promoting the concept that, following divorce or separation, mothers and fathers should retain a strong positive parenting role with the children spending substantial amounts of time living with each parent.)
www.spig.clara.net

The Single and Custodial Father's Network
(A US-based online support and networking organisation)
www.scfn.org

Single Parent Action Network UK
(Provides information, advice and support to one parent families)
Tel: 0117 951 4231
www.spanuk.org.uk

Stay at home dads
(Provides information and support for househusbands - US-based)
www.slowlane.com

Stonewall
(Advice, information and support for gay parents)
www.stonewall.org.uk

ukparents.co.uk
(An information and community service, mainly aimed at mothers but with useful information for dads too)
www.ukparents.co.uk

Name / organisation	Address	Telephone	Next appointment
GP			
Hospital			
Dentist			
Optician			

National insurance number . . . .

Private health insurance number . . . .

Blood group . . . .

Height . . . .

Actual weight . . . .

Target weight . . . .

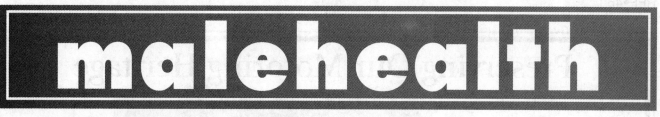

malehealth

a unique health website

fast, free independent info from the Men's Health Forum

Want to find out more?

malehealth.co.uk is a new health website aimed at blokes of all ages - it aims to bring you the information you want in a form that's easy to read and even easier to find.

At its heart is a Key Info section which covers 24 common health topics in a clear Q and A format. It includes, for beginners, the Male Body - A User's Guide, an overview of every part of the male anatomy.

You can get an instant online health report and we'll talk you through how to do a home MOT health check. Then there's frank healthy living advice in the Easy Ways to Feel Better section including all our favourite subjects: drink, smoking, sex, food and exercise. And, for those who want a more detailed work-out, there is our online gym including a seven week fitness programme specially designed by Britain's most capped athlete. On top of all that, there's news, features, statistics and links to useful books and other web-sites.

Register for a free newsletter to get all the latest updates. It all adds up to a very comprehensive site - so far as we know, the only one of its type in the world.

The site is run by the Men's Health Forum, the leading voluntary organisation working to improve men's health in the UK, of which Dr Ian Banks is president. So take Dr Ian's advice: prescribe yourself a visit to malehealth today.

Look forward to seeing you,

Jim Pollard, editor, malehealth.co.uk

www.malehealth.co.uk

Preserving Our Motoring Heritage

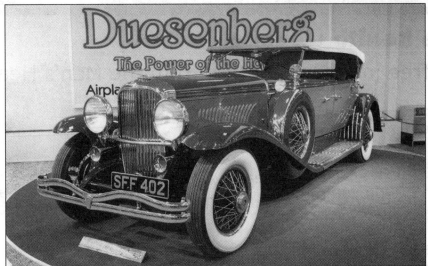

> <
> *The Model J Duesenberg Derham Tourster. Only eight of these magnificent cars were ever built – this is the only example to be found outside the United States of America*

Almost every car you've ever loved, loathed or desired is gathered under one roof at the Haynes Motor Museum. Over 300 immaculately presented cars and motorbikes represent every aspect of our motoring heritage, from elegant reminders of bygone days, such as the superb Model J Duesenberg to curiosities like the bug-eyed BMW Isetta. There are also many old friends and flames. Perhaps you remember the 1959 Ford Popular that you did your courting in? The magnificent 'Red Collection' is a spectacle of classic sports cars including AC, Alfa Romeo, Austin Healey, Ferrari, Lamborghini, Maserati, MG, Riley, Porsche and Triumph.

A Perfect Day Out

Each and every vehicle at the Haynes Motor Museum has played its part in the history and culture of Motoring. Today, they make a wonderful spectacle and a great day out for all the family. Bring the kids, bring Mum and Dad, but above all bring your camera to capture those golden memories for ever. You will also find an impressive array of motoring memorabilia, a comfortable 70 seat video cinema and one of the most extensive transport book shops in Britain. The Pit Stop Cafe serves everything from a cup of tea to wholesome, home-made meals or, if you prefer, you can enjoy the large picnic area nestled in the beautiful rural surroundings of Somerset.

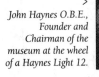

> *John Haynes O.B.E., Founder and Chairman of the museum at the wheel of a Haynes Light 12.*

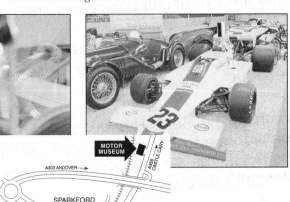

> <
> *Graham Hill's Lola Cosworth Formula 1 car next to a 1934 Riley Sports.*

The Museum is situated on the A359 Yeovil to Frome road at Sparkford, just off the A303 in Somerset. It is about 40 miles south of Bristol, and 25 minutes drive from the M5 intersection at Taunton.

Open 9.30am - 5.30pm (10.00am - 4.00pm Winter) 7 days a week, *except Christmas Day, Boxing Day and New Years Day*

Special rates available for schools, coach parties and outings Charitable Trust No. 292048